Comments on *Migraine* from a reader

'This very interesting book has filled in lots of gaps for me –
about the causes of migraine headaches and about the different
sorts of treatment. It will help me to prevent attacks and, when
one occurs, will help me to treat it more effectively.'

Judith Wise, London

Migraine

Practical advice to help you manage your migraine

F. Clifford Rose MD, FRCP

*Director and Consultant Neurologist,
London Neurological Centre;
Honorary Consulting Neurologist,
Charing Cross Hospital;
Trustee, The Migraine Trust*

and

Marek Gawel MA, MB BCh, FRCP (UK), FRCPC

*Director, Headache Research Unit, Sunnybrook
and Women's Health Sciences Centre, Toronto*

Class Publishing • London

Printing history
First published as *Migraine: the facts* by Oxford University Press 1979
This fully revised edition first published 2004

The authors and publisher welcome feedback from the users of
this book. Please contact the publisher.
**Class Publishing, Barb House, Barb Mews, London W6 7PA, UK
Telephone: 020 7371 2119   Fax: 020 7371 2878 [International +4420]
email: post@class.co.uk
Visit our website – www.class.co.uk**

The information presented in this book is accurate and current to the
best of the authors' knowledge. The authors and publisher, however,
make no guarantee as to, and assume no responsibility for, the
correctness, sufficiency or completeness of such information or
recommendation. The reader is advised to consult a doctor regarding
all aspects of individual health care.

A CIP catalogue for this book is available from the British Library.

ISBN 1 85959 066 7

Contents

Foreword

As a migraine sufferer who heads an organisation dedicated to funding research into the causes and treatment of migraine, which also engages on a day-to-day basis with sufferers and their carers, I am acutely aware of the desire for up-to-date, accurate information. In this greatly enhanced edition of their original classic reference, aimed at the general public, Dr Frank Clifford Rose and Dr Marek Gawel enable those affected by migraine and other debilitating headaches to better understand their condition and treatments.

Whether you are looking for greater understanding of migraine, information on treatment with or without drugs, or confirmation that your migraine is being appropriately managed, I highly recommend this book. Without doubt the authors have successfully written from immense medical background and knowledge in a way that will be easily comprehended by a lay audience, although I believe that many in the medical profession will also find this work an invaluable resource.

Migraine may not be life-threatening but both sufferers and their families can have their lives greatly disrupted by this debilitating condition. I hope that many will find themselves informed, and therefore empowered, by this book to the point where they take control and better manage their migraine.

ALAN BARTLE
Chief Executive,
The Migraine Trust

1
What is migraine?

The word 'migraine' comes from the Greek term for a one-sided headache (*hemi-crania*). But not all headaches are due to migraine and, because the treatment will depend on the cause, it is important to separate the different types of headache. Various types of migrainous headaches are described in this chapter, and in Chapter 2 we discuss some headaches that are not migraine. Headaches that are the result of trauma, such as a road traffic accident, are discussed in Chapter 3.

Migraine is not a trivial disorder, because the problems it poses to the people affected, their families, their work and social life can be enormous. Interest in the subject is increasing dramatically, partly because of a growing awareness of the disability caused by migraine, partly because of the rapid growth in knowledge of the condition but more significantly because of newer effective treatments. Another factor is the support of the pharmaceutical industry, which sees the widespread need for effective drugs to treat or prevent migraine attacks.

The brain

The involvement of the brain in migraine is discussed fully in Chapter 6. Now, however, it is useful to outline the structure of the brain and its role in our senses.

The brain is made up of four lobes (Figure 1.1):

- one in the front (the frontal lobe),
- one at the back (the occipital lobe),
- one in between (the parietal lobe), and
- one below (the temporal lobe).

The occipital lobe is where vision takes place, especially in the visual cortex. The flickering blurred vision of the migraine warning comes from the grey matter of the occipital cortex. The cortex is the outside of the whole brain (grey matter) and consists of the cell bodies of neurones (nerve cells). The white matter, which forms the inside of the brain, is made up of the nerve fibres, which come from the cell bodies and join with other cells

The parietal lobe governs movement, the frontal lobe sensation and personality, while the temporal lobe serves memory functions. The language centre is the back part of the dominant temporal lobe which, in over 90 per cent of people, is on the left side.

The brain consists of 10–100 *billion* nerve cells (neurones). Each neurone consists of a cell body, which contains the nucleus, which governs the electrical messages that are conducted along the nerve fibres. All nerve cells are connected to other cells by

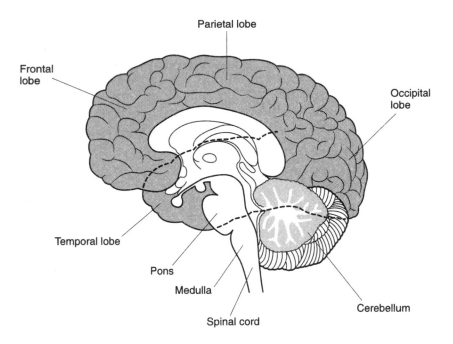

Figure 1.1 The main parts of the brain, including the four lobes (viewed from the side).

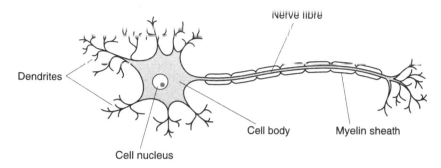

Figure 1.2 A nerve cell

chemical 'messengers' called neurotransmitters. Unlike the cells in peripheral nerves, the neurones of the central nervous system (brain and spinal cord) do not regenerate. Although we lose about 100,000 cells every day from the age of 18, we have actually lost only about 3 per cent of our brain cells by the time we are 70, and experience more than makes up for this loss.

Migraine with aura

This type of migraine used to be called 'classic migraine', because it was easily recognised, suggesting in some way that this was the fully developed form. It is true, however, that most people have migraine without the aura – the so-called 'common migraine'. The new terminology – 'migraine with aura' and 'migraine without aura' came into effect in 1988 when the classification committee of the International Headache Society published the *Classification of headache disorders, cranial neuralgias and facial pain.* Although this has become the standard for diagnosis, at least for the research purposes for which it was designed, many people stick to 'classic' and 'common' for everyday purposes.

The description of typical, common, migraine includes three features:

- it is one-sided,
- it is accompanied by nausea and sometimes vomiting,
- there is sensitivity to light and/or sound and/or smell.

In classic migraine there is, in addition, the warning – or aura – most often from disturbance of vision.

The following description comes from Angela Baker, a 32-year-old social worker.

> *I wake up in the morning feeling happy. The sky seems more blue – in fact, all colours appear more intense. I know this means that later that day, or perhaps the next, I will get a migraine attack. The pain gradually comes on over one temple, usually the right, and spreads over the whole of that side of my head. At the same time, but sometimes before the headache begins, part of my vision blurs, bright 'stars' may appear and move over my field of vision. The headache becomes worse and throbbing, I start feeling sick. If I vomit, this seems to make the headache better. With the headache, light hurts my eyes so I have to go to bed after drawing the curtains. The whole attack lasts about eight hours and leaves me tired and shaky.*

This is a description of an attack of *migraine with aura*, or *classic migraine*. In addition to the four classic features (one-sided headache, nausea and vomiting, sensitivity to light and/or sound, and visual disturbances), it includes other characteristics found with migrainous attacks.

The warning – the premonitory phase

The warning of several hours, or a day or even two, before the actual attack is well known to many people with migraine. Although in Angela's case it took the form of feeling happy and being more aware of colours, there may be other variations in mood, increased energy, a feeling of hunger or thirst, or even just the feeling that something is about to happen. When hunger is the warning, over-eating can sometimes prevent the attack. A craving for chocolate is quite common, which may be why some people believe that eating chocolate triggers a migraine, although in fact it doesn't but coincides with the beginning of an attack.

The warning period probably stems from a chemical imbalance in the areas of the brain that control mood and emotion. One such area at the base of the brain, the *hypo-thalamus*, controls the secretion of several hormones and it is possible that an alteration in its normal functioning may be a trigger for the headache that follows. One neurotransmitter (a chemical 'messenger' between nerve cells) is dopamine; as this may be involved in the warning part of the attack, taking an anti dopamine drug (e.g. domperidone) at this stage can abort the attack.

Aura

Although the premonitory symptoms can last 24 hours or more, the next phase – the aura itself – is much shorter, the visual aura lasting only 20–30 minutes. Other symptoms can include such neurological symptoms as confusion, inability to concentrate, problems with co-ordination and slurred speech.

Blurred vision is frequent but the most characteristic visual symptom is an inability to see part of the visual field (the area being looked at). The visual abnormalities can take different forms and be very dramatic (see Figures 1.3 to 1.9). One side of the visual field may be fragmented and interrupted by shiny lines, arranged like constellations, a phenomenon known as *fortification spectra*, because of its resemblance to a castellated fort. Some mystics have interpreted these as visions of, for example, 'the eternal city'. Another term for this type of visual

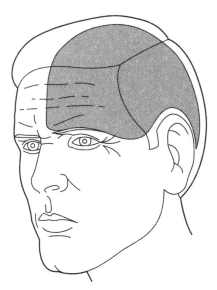

Figure 1.3 Migraine with aura (classic migraine): an aura is usually present before the headache begins

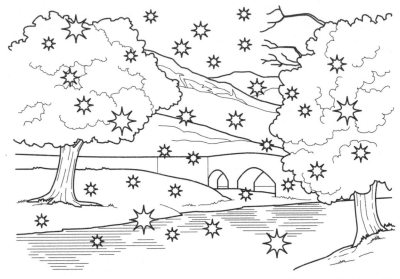

Figure 1.4 Bright shimmering 'stars' seen falling across the image (teichopsia)

aura is *teichopsia* (*teichos* being the Greek word for a wall). There may also be small multicoloured areas of flashing lights,

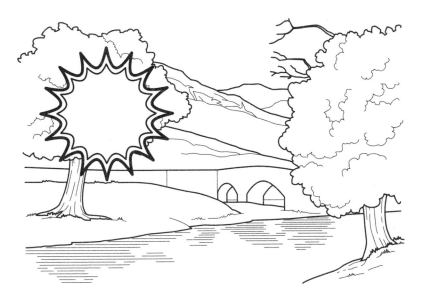

Figure 1.5 Scintillating scotoma: an area of loss of vision surrounded by a bright starburst; this often moves across the field of vision

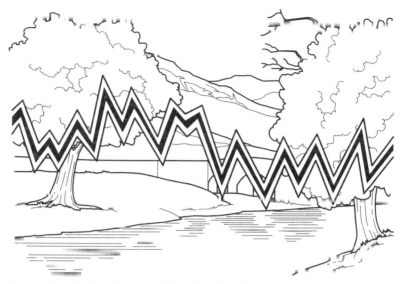

Figure 1.6 Bright-edged, castellated line (fortification spectrum or teichopsia)

zigzag patterns or 'Catherine wheels', and there is usually generalised blurring of vision, as if looking through steam or

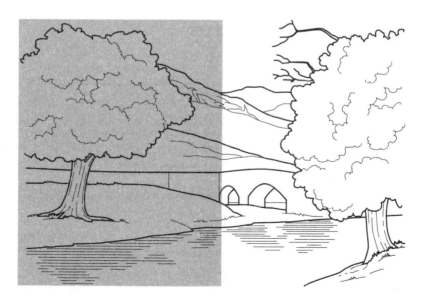

Figure 1.7 Loss, blanking or darkening of one half of the field of vision (hemianopia)

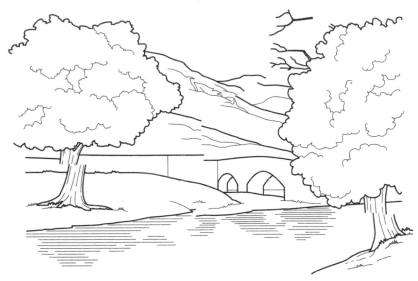

Figure 1.8 Fragmentation of the visual image

water. Another common visual feature is the loss of vision either in a roughly semicircular area or in half of the visual field, i.e. the

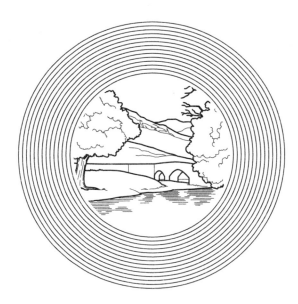

Figure 1.9 Tunnel vision. The visual image appears smaller and more distant, as if viewed down the wrong end of a telescope

area seen to one side. One side of the body is controlled by the opposite half (hemispheric) of the brain, so the area perceived on one side is a function of the opposite side of the brain; this means that damage to the visual area (occipital cortex) of the left half of the brain produces a loss in vision of the right half of the visual field in *both* eyes. Such a blanking-out during a migraine attack indicates that one hemisphere of the brain is affected, but only temporarily.

Less common disturbances of perception are changes in the size and the shape of objects, objects seeming to be tilted or far away, or that colours have faded. (These effects are due to changes in function of the parietal lobes of the brain, which deal with orientation in space and time.)

People having a migraine attack sometimes complain that they feel taller, or, conversely, are 'about one foot high'. At one time it was thought that Lewis Carroll, a migraine sufferer, was drawing on his own experience of such sensations in *Alice in Wonderland*, but this intriguing explanation was somewhat discredited by his diary, which suggests that he wrote the book *before* he developed migrainous symptoms.

The visual disturbances usually herald the onset of headache but occasionally occur later in the attack. Rarely, the headache itself plays only a small part in the attack, when it is called *acephalgic migraine* (i.e. migraine without headache). The following case history demonstrates this.

> *Charles Dodds, a 42-year-old physician, was driving along Regent Street, London, during the rush-hour to an appointment for which he was late. He suddenly found he could not read the number-plate of the car immediately in front of him. He had never before suffered from migrainous symptoms. After about 30 seconds the blind spot (scotoma) began to alter, opening up to form an enlarging crescent of shimmering angles that spread to the periphery of his visual field and disappeared. This phenomenon – a typical migrainous aura – lasted precisely 20 minutes and was followed by irritability and lack of appetite lasting a few hours, but he had no headache.*

There is little doubt that these symptoms were migrainous in origin despite the absence of headache. The cause of such an attack may be a change of electrical conductivity (called 'spreading depression') rather than a narrowing of blood vessels (vasoconstriction) feeding the brain.

Other manifestations include temporary weakness and numbness of the arm and face on one side (*hemiplegic migraine*, discussed below). The weakness, which can be as severe as that occurring in stroke, may continue after the headache has gone. There is an inherited form of migraine called *familial hemiplegic migraine* in which the person becomes paralysed down one side during attacks. This form runs in families and the gene responsible for it has been located on chromosome 19.

Other people with migraine report changes in their hearing; for instance, speech may sound like a recording that is being played at too fast a speed. Sounds may seem overwhelmingly loud (*hyperacusis*) or even upsetting (*phonophobia*), or continue to reverberate after they have ceased. Rarely, it may seem that there is another person looking on – the *doppelgänger*.

People who have migraine may not mention such odd sensations and perceptions for fear of being thought insane but all these phenomena are consistent with a migrainous aura.

Migraine without aura

Only a minority of people with migraine (about 10 per cent) have an aura or other brain features described above.

The headache

Pain over one temple is usually the first sign, followed by pain over the same side of the head (see Figure 1.3). The pain often spreads to the whole of the head. Often the headache is not one-sided, or may be one-sided at first and then moves around the head during the attack and then becomes generalised. The pain is due to the release of chemical messengers from the nerve termi-nals around the blood vessels, which alter their sensitivity and size. These messengers are released by signals travelling to the nerve terminals from the governing body (the nucleus) of the trigeminal nerve, which carries sensation from the head and face to the brain. We know from recent research that the stimulus takes place in the brain stem (hypothalamus). The characteristic throbbing sensation is due to the pulse pounding against these dilated sensitive blood vessels. The headache can last as long as 24 hours (officially from 4 to 72 hours) but is generally no more than six to eight hours (as with Angela Baker); sometimes the person having an attack is lucky enough to be able to fall asleep, and may discover on waking that the pain has gone.

It is very common during a migraine headache to find light troublesome and disturbing (photophobia) whereas darkness is soothing.

There are other types of headache that are also included under the umbrella term of migraine but they differ from classic or common migraine in several respects.

Basilar migraine

This rare form usually occurs in children. The headache is commonly over the back of the head and, besides nausea, the symptoms may include double vision, giddiness, unsteadiness and slurred speech. Perhaps the most alarming symptom is loss of consciousness. These symptoms are due to a disturbance of that part of the brain (the brain stem) supplied by the basilar artery.

Hemiplegic migraine

This is a very rare form in which there is paralysis of the arm and leg on one side of the body. Fortunately, the paralysis is temporary but it may recur. There is sometimes a strong family history of similar attacks – familial hemiplegic migraine. As mentioned earlier, the gene for this latter form has been identified on chromosome 19; the gene is that part of a chromosome found in the cell nucleus that governs the function of a cell.

The covering of a cell, the cell membrane, has microscopic pores called channels, which control the flow of certain ions (electrically charged pairs of molecules). It is through these that changes in ionic flow occur (e.g. calcium ions in a *calcium channel*). These channels control the flow of certain ions that generate electrical charges which produce the impulses that travel down the nerves; the relevant gene may be responsible for a change in the flow of ions, which predisposes to migraine.

Ophthalmoplegic migraine

This is rare, and occurs particularly in children. During or following an attack, one eyelid droops, the pupil on that side enlarges (dilates) and the eye squints outward. As with other types of migraine, these features are temporary and usually go when the headache stops. More often than not, this type of migraine often has an underlying cause (e.g. inflammation or a cyst behind the eye) and therefore needs investigating.

Abdominal migraine

This occurs more commonly in childhood. The pain, which lasts a few hours, is often over the upper part of the abdomen. The diagnosis is suggested by the family history of migraine and some attacks in which the pain is accompanied by about an hour of typical migraine headache. There may be associated nausea and vomiting that recurs (cyclical vomiting). Any of these features in children can presage migraine later in life, as does easily induced travel sickness.

Facial migraine

Some people feel the pain of migraine in the face, either in a distribution in and around the eye or lower down the cheek. In these cases the pain is less severe, less sharp and may last for much longer than in a migraine attack with or without aura.

Chronic daily headache

One of the most difficult problems facing a family doctor is the person who has very frequent headaches. These patients often complain that they have a headache nearly every day, the severity varying but some regularly being very much worse. There does not seem to be any particular trigger for these headaches – they just come. They can be extremely debilitating, rendering people completely unfit for any occupation and making them unable to function socially.

In the past, one of the causes of 'chronic daily headache' was over-use of ergotamine to treat migraine; people using ergotamine this way eventually developed what was then called *chronic ergotamine overuse headache*. They would wake up in the morning with a headache, having used ergotamine the day before for a previous headache. Basically this was a form of 'rebound' in that the headache which had been suppressed yesterday began again when the ergotamine wore off. It is now known that almost any analgesic (pain-killer) can cause this sort of headache, called *analgesic headache* (or *medication overuse headache* or *medication-induced headache*).

Because people with migraine often go through periods when their headaches become more frequent, more and more pain-killers are used in order to get them through the day. The headaches eventually become almost continuous and so medication is taken all the time in order to function. Ultimately, the pain-killer ceases to be effective and headaches occur daily. The treatment for this is for the person to understand what has happened and stop using the pain-killers. This can be very difficult for people, because, when they stop taking the medication, they get an even worse headache for a few days; some of them may need to be admitted to a hospital or clinic to wean them off the offending medication. Preventive medication can sometimes be helpful.

One method, or protocol, developed in North America is to admit the individual to hospital for a few days for dihydroergotamine to be given intravenously. After the offending medication is stopped, dihydroergotamine is given several times a day until the patient improves. Strict follow-up is necessary because there is a return to the previous situation in nearly half the people treated this way.

Those who continue to have daily headaches despite stopping all their pain-killers may have a tension-type headache (see Chapter 2) or be at the extreme end of the migraine continuum; they constitute about 5 per cent of the whole migraine population. Here, the use of a triptan (see Chapter 9) may help but the headache can return as soon as the triptan wears off. Some individuals may end up taking a triptan daily, which is not advisable, and referral to a headache specialist is then required.

Many people who attend a headache clinic suffer from chronic daily headaches. Their management consists of a judicious mix of advice, non-drug therapy (discussed in Chapter 8) and preventive drugs (discussed in Chapter 9), as well as tablets to treat symptoms. Because these patients become increasingly desperate, it is important to help them understand the nature of their condition by building a good and trustful relationship between doctor and patient. The doctor must not be judgmental, because medication-induced headaches have altered the patient's body responses.

Mrs Greta Winfield, a 46-year-old nurse, had suffered from migraine for most of her life. The headaches would usually come around her periods. They would be associated with nausea and sensitivity to light and sound. Occasionally, about 20 minutes before the headache, she would see a shimmering pattern in front of her eyes – which would disappear as the headache started. The headaches would last about six hours but responded to treatment with either simple pain-killers or a triptan. A year previously she had gone on night shift, which resulted in disrupted sleep. Her headaches became more frequent so, in order to maintain her efficiency at work, she began to take an over-the-counter (no prescription needed) combination of paracetamol and codeine in increasingly large amounts. Gradually the headaches became more and more frequent, necessitating large amounts of pain-killer.

When she was seen at the headache clinic she was having daily headaches. Twice a week they were so bad, with vomiting and consequent dehydration, that they would barely respond to any treatment; she would have to leave work early because she was unable to carry out many of her duties. Her periods had become more irregular. Being unfit to work, she was becoming increasingly desperate.

The physical examination was normal, as was neurological testing and a CT scan of the brain. It is important to have a CT (computed tomography) scan or, preferably, MRI (magnetic resonance imaging) if the nature of the headaches has changed, to exclude the possibility of a more serious cause for them.

She was admitted to hospital and was given dihydro-ergotamine and metoclopramide intravenously three times a day for four days. All her pain-killers were stopped; she was started on preventive medication and her headaches subsided. She was taught how to inject dihydroergotamine and continued to do this as necessary at home. Subsequently the medication was changed to a triptan (see Chapter 9), which managed to control her headaches well. At follow-up, she was getting only one headache every three or four weeks, which was easily controllable.

This case illustrates what we understand to be medication-induced headache. A variety of factors such as sleep deprivation, change in working hours and fluctuations in hormonal state had all come together to increase the frequency of headaches. Taking increasing amounts of pain-killers aggravated the situation, producing chronic daily headache.

George Campbell, a 34-year-old man, woke up one morning with a headache: it was one-sided, throbbing, and associated with mild nausea and some sensitivity to light. He improved with pain-killers but the headache returned when the pain-killers had worn off. The headache persisted and at the time of his visit to the headache clinic he'd had it for six months non-stop. At times it would improve slightly, with less throbbing or light sensitivity, but at other times it would get even worse. Although responding temporarily to treatment, it would always come back.

Investigations included blood tests, MRI and a lumbar puncture (spinal tap) to monitor his spinal fluid pressure. None of them showed any reason for this continued headache.

Methods of treatment of this chronic daily headache are not always successful. The preventive medication is given as for any other migraine attack as well as appropriate drugs to treat the symptoms but avoiding the trap of developing *super-added medication-induced headache.*

2
Other headaches

Tension-type headaches

These headaches used to be called *tension headache* or *muscle-contraction headache* but the names were changed by the International Headache Society's classification to *tension-type headaches*. One reason for this change was the problem of whether the word 'tension' referred to tension in the muscles or psychological tension; another was to emphasise that they are not all caused by muscle contraction. Tightening of the muscles at the back of the neck has been blamed as causing tension of the scalp (see Figure 2.1). The pain can be felt at the back of the

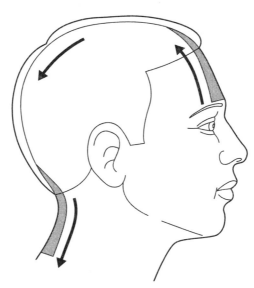

Figure 2.1 Muscle-contraction (tension) headache: the muscles at the back of the neck become tense, pulling on the scalp and stretching the forehead muscles

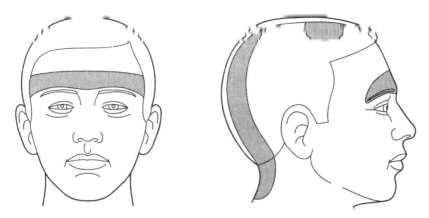

Figure 2.2 Tension-type headache: the headache is felt like a tight band round the head; the pain may also be felt in the back of the neck and on top of the head

neck, over the top of the head or over the forehead, and is often described as a 'vice round the head' (see Figure 2.2). Tension in the muscles may be painful in itself, but associated constriction of the arteries within the muscles has been suggested as making the pain considerably worse. The electromyograph (EMG) uses a machine that measures electrical activity as a sign of muscle contraction, which can occur excessively during this form of headache, although not always.

Tension-type headache not associated with muscle contraction is possibly caused by the brain mis-sensing nerve impulses arriving from the head and labelling them as painful. This type of tension-type headache has the same symptoms as those associated with muscle contraction – probably because the same pathways are used for the pain messages despite their different origins.

Georgina Holmes, a 45-year-old housewife, said:

> *For the past nine months I have had almost continuous headaches. It is as if I have a heavy weight on the top of my head. I notice it as soon as I wake in the morning and it lasts all day. It does not keep me awake at night but it is there when I wake up in the morning. I do not feel sick and have no trouble with my eyes. Sometimes I feel a tight band around my head and usually the back of my neck feels stiff.*

This is a typical tension-type headache, which may or may not be associated with muscle contraction, as shown by electrical activity on the electromyograph. When Georgina was questioned, she revealed that the headaches had started after a particularly stressful argument with her teenage daughter. This type of headache can be due to depression, particularly when associated with early-morning waking, feelings of apathy and not wanting to do anything. These headaches can be improved considerably by drugs called tricyclics. In large doses (100–150mg) tricyclics are given as antidepressants but in smaller daily doses (10–25mg at night) they are highly effective for these headaches. Care should be taken with the newer antidepressants, the specific serotonin reuptake inhibitors (SSRIs), because they can cause increased frequency and severity of headache.

Tension-type headache is more common than migraine but the two types can often occur together in the same person – a condition called *combined headaches*. Although tension-type headache in people without migraine does not respond to migraine-specific drugs, it may do so if migraine *is* present. This suggests that the accompanying so-called tension-type headache might be a minor form (*forme fruste*) of migraine.

Cluster headache

Edward Finlay, a 35-year-old financial adviser, described an attack as follows:

> *I am woken in the early hours of the morning by an intense pain behind my left eye, as if someone was sticking a red-hot needle into it. I get out of bed to find that my nose feels blocked and my left eye is watering. When I look in the mirror, the eye is red. The attack lasts half an hour and goes as quickly as it came. The extraordinary thing is that the attack occurs every night at around 2 to 3 a.m. and this has been going on for nearly three weeks.*

This is a typical example of *cluster headache* (previously called *migrainous neuralgia* although it is neither migraine nor neuralgia). Men are affected more often than women (at a rate of about 6:1) and it usually starts between the ages of 30 and 50, which is a later onset than with migraine. They are often woken at night by a severe pain behind one eye – nearly always the

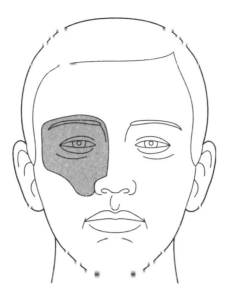

Figure 2.3 Cluster headache: the severe pain is felt behind one eye, nearly always the same eye

same eye – often described as crushing, like a 'hot poker', or stabbing (Figure 2.3). There is often watering of the affected eye, which is reddened, and the nostril on that side becomes stuffy, blocked and may even run. The attack may last for about an hour and then go, only to return the following night at the same time. During an attack the upper eyelid on the affected side may droop, and the pupil on that side becomes smaller than the pupil on the normal side. The episodes last several weeks and, for this reason, they are called 'cluster headaches' but there are nearly 20 other names. The cluster may occur two or three times a year or only once in two or three years. The following case history demonstrates these points.

Will Xerxes, a 50-year-old man about 1.9m (6ft 3in) tall and weighing 95kg (15 stone), was under a good deal of pressure at work and was also active as secretary of a number of voluntary organisations. One Christmas, he began to have attacks of severe pain behind the right eye, which went red, and his right nostril became blocked. The pain woke him and lasted for half an hour. He was unable to go to sleep again and was becoming increasingly tired.

The initial treatment was zolmitriptan (Zomig) three times daily for a limited period to try to break the pattern, but to no avail. It was then decided to try steroids, and he took prednisolone three times daily. This form of treatment can be used for only a short time and the course was stopped three weeks later; he was free of headaches for three weeks, at which point they returned. He then tried verapamil, a calcium blocker, and the headaches came under good control.

The 'periodicity' of these attacks has puzzled scientists for many years. Someone who used to have attacks every Christmas decided to avoid them by spending Christmas in Australia; the attacks came just the same!

During an attack a technique called positron emission tomography (PET) reveals that there is an area of the brain which becomes activated. How it happens is another matter but it is this part of the brain that controls biological cycles and body rhythms. Called the lateral hypothalamus, it is larger in people with cluster headaches as shown on MRI than in those who do not have them.

Inflammatory diseases

When micro-organisms invade the body, a battle ensues between them and the body's defences. White blood cells are mobilised and some of them release active substances – neurotransmitters – into the local circulation. A similar release of active substances occurs during allergic reactions or when a weal or blister from a burn forms on the skin. These substances cause increased sensitivity to pain. They are divided into two groups: *kinins*, which are derived from the breakdown of protein; and *amines* – especially *histamine*, which causes more inflammation and makes the blood vessels porous, producing swelling and redness. Other neurotransmitters also play a part in inflammation, and include the prostaglandins and leukotrienes.

Sinusitis

Infection in the sinuses gives rise to sinusitis (the 'itis' means inflammation, so 'sinusitis' means inflammation in the sinus(es)).

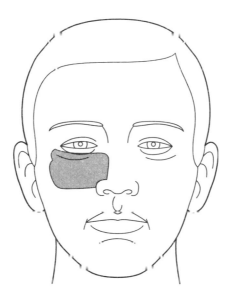

Figure 2.4 Sinusitis: pain over the affected (maxillary) sinus

The pain of sinusitis tends to affect the area either above the eye (the frontal sinus) or below it (the maxillary sinus) (see Figure 2.4). The pain often comes on after a cold that blocks the nose, and occurs every day – being worse in the afternoons. It is the result of inflammation and stretching of the lining of the sinus (mucous membrane) and the layer of tissue covering the bone (periosteum); the blood vessels are distended and fluids (oedema) are produced by any inflammation. The affected area is often tender to pressure or tapping, and the diagnosis of sinusitis can be confirmed by X-rays, CT or MRI.

The treatment consists of antibiotics and drainage of fluid and pus from the infected sinus. When the condition is recurrent or protracted, surgical therapy is sometimes indicated.

Meningitis

This is an inflammation of the brain's coverings (the meninges) and always includes headache. The intense pain in the head is associated with contraction of the neck muscles, which produces a stiff neck – a typical symptom of meningitis. It is a serious condition and, when suspected, a spinal tap (lumbar puncture) is necessary to examine the cerebrospinal fluid for evidence of infection or inflammation, and to try to determine the organism causing the problem.

Some types of infection are more dangerous than others, but even the worst can usually be cured by modern antibiotics, particularly if the diagnosis is made early.

Encephalitis

This is inflammation of the brain, and is another very serious cause of headache. It is most often caused by viruses and, because of this, is not easily treatable. Some forms of encephalitis are found in particular areas of the world; for example, Eastern Equine Encephalitis which occurs on the east coast of North America.

One previously lethal form caused by the virus *Herpes simplex* is now treatable with the antiviral drug aciclovir or its more modern forms.

Dental infection

This is sometimes a cause of headache but is more likely to cause pain in the jaws – the lower jaw being affected more commonly than the upper. When this is suspected, the individual should be referred to a dentist.

Less common causes of headache

Trigeminal neuralgia

This affects people in the second half of life, women twice as often as men. It consists of paroxysms of severe shooting or stabbing pains on one side of the face (Figure 2.5), which are brought on by eating, talking, cold draughts, cleaning teeth or, in men, shaving. The painful spasms may last only a few seconds but can recur frequently.

The treatment is usually effective with the drug carbamazepine; if this doesn't work, the neuralgia may respond to other drugs such as phenytoin, gabapentin or topiramate (anti-

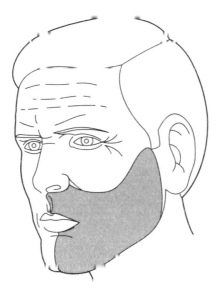

Figure 2.5 Trigeminal neuralgia: the stabbing pain may affect any part of the face but is usually in the lower parts (the mandibular and/or maxillary division of the trigeminal nerve, which supplies sensation to one side of the face)

epilepsy drugs). In cases that are very resistant, a direct attack on part of the nerve (the trigeminal ganglion) may be necessary – by injection, laser therapy or surgery.

The cervical spine

Abnormalities of the bones in the neck – the cervical spine – are often said to be the cause of headache but this is much less common than is supposed. An X-ray of anyone over the age of 50 years may reveal changes in the cervical spine but this does not necessarily mean they are the cause of the headaches.

Nevertheless, when the neck *is* the cause of the headache and anti-inflammatory drugs have failed, treatment is aimed at removing the source of irritation. To do this, diagnostic 'blocks' of joints that link the vertebrae (facet joints) are performed: the nerves at various levels in the neck are 'frozen' with local anaesthetic. If the pain is relieved temporarily, the area can be cauterised using a microwave probe to destroy the nerves at each level. In this procedure a needle containing a microwave electrode is inserted next to the nerve, under X-ray control, and a current passed. The nerve carrying the impulses is destroyed and blocks the painful stimuli. It causes no lasting problems and although sensation may be affected initially, it returns within six months.

Food

There are many other less common causes of headache that come on after eating certain foods that are not migrainous or allergic in type but to which the person has a sensitivity. The headaches will pass after a time, and susceptible people learn to avoid the 'trigger' foods (see Chapter 6).

The 'Chinese restaurant' syndrome

The symptoms develop within half an hour of starting a Chinese meal. Although one feature is headache, affecting chiefly the temples and forehead, the chief complaints are a feeling of tightness or pressure over the face and chest, with flushing and sweating of the face.

The offending substance is the chemical monosodium glutamate (MSG). This is added to food to bring out its taste, and is regularly used in Chinese food. Just 3 grams of MSG is enough to bring on the symptoms in susceptible people, particularly if taken on an empty stomach. The syndrome is therefore more likely to occur after soup, when absorption of the substance is more rapid, than after more solid food.

Hot-dog (or cured meat) headache

Some people complain of headaches after eating cured meats, of which hot-dog sausage is a classic example; others include bacon, ham and salami. The headache starts within half an hour of eating these foods. The offending substances are nitrites, which are added to the salt used in the curing process in order to give the meats a uniform red colour. Both nitrates and nitrites are well known vasodilators (i.e. they widen the blood vessels), producing flushing of the face.

Nitric oxide is one of the transmitters within the nervous system, which play a part in vasodilatation. Attempts to block the activity of nitric oxide synthetase is now being tried to treat or prevent migraine attacks. A drug used for erectile dysfunction, sildenafil (Viagra), acts by increasing blood flow to specific areas in the body; it has the occasional side-effect of headache because it increases the amount of nitric oxide available.

Ice-cream headache

This headache is caused by having very cold substances such as ice or ice-cream in the mouth. The intense cooling of the roof of the mouth produces a pain that is then 'referred' to the head. This type of headache can be prevented if the ice-cream is taken slowly. When it happens in migraine, it often affects the side where the migraine occurs most frequently.

Alcohol

Alcohol is a powerful vasodilator, as can be seen from the flushed face of someone who has drunk too much. Headache can develop when the alcohol is being drunk but the term 'hangover' is restricted to the symptoms – of which headache is predominant – that occur several hours later, usually the next day. This is due to the breakdown products when alcohol is metabolised, and includes such substances as acetates and acetaldehyde. Alcohol causes an increase in passing urine (diuresis), resulting in dehydration, so drinking a lot of water helps to prevent the symptoms of a hangover.

Exertional headache

With exercise, muscles require more blood and so their blood vessels widen (dilate) to help the circulation. This is why faces become flushed during exercise. The blood pressure also changes and this, with further stretching of the dilated intracranial blood vessels, can cause headache. These 'exertional' headaches are very occasionally due to an underlying problem, so further investigation may be required to rule out any alteration of brain structure.

Headache associated with sexual intercourse is an example of exercise headache. It occurs at or near the time of orgasm and can be very severe. Although the pain usually lasts only a few minutes, it can persist after intercourse and last for days. It affects women as well as men, and can occur with masturbation. The blood pressure can rise more than 50 per cent and the pulse rate double during intercourse, so it is surprising that this type of headache is not more common.

Extremely rarely, an intense headache may be caused by a bleed from a weakened blood vessel that balloons out to become an *aneurysm*. Although migraine is also caused by exertion or intercourse, when these headaches keep recurring, it is advisable to seek medical attention so that any underlying other cause can be ruled out.

High blood pressure

Probably the most common cause of headache in people with high blood pressure (hypertension) is anxiety about their blood pressure. But there is no doubt that marked ('malignant') hypertension can cause severe headache along with other neurological disturbances (*hypertensive encephalopathy*). People with both migraine and high blood pressure often find that, when the blood pressure is brought down to normal levels, the intensity and frequency of the migraine attacks lessen.

Strokes

There are two main types of stroke, depending on whether the blood vessel to the brain bleeds (*cerebral haemorrhage*) or is blocked (*cerebral infarction*). People with cerebral haemorrhage nearly always have a headache, particularly if the blood gets into the space surrounding the brain (*subarachnoid haemorrhage*). This bleeding often arises from a weakened part of a blood vessel that has ballooned out, forming an aneurysm, or occasionally from an abnormal group of blood vessels – an *angioma* or *arteriovenus malformation*). Whatever the cause, the symptoms are usually typical: a sudden pain is felt at the back of or across the head as if the person had been struck with a hammer; loss of consciousness may follow. The headache persists and the irritation of the meninges causes symptoms resembling meningitis (see above).

Temporal arteritis

With this condition the arteries in the temples are more thickened and tortuous, and they are particularly tender because they are inflamed. This produces a very severe headache in people over the age of 55 years, and usually much older. Someone with temporal arteritis is generally unwell and may have had pains all over the body (polymyalgia rheumatica) for weeks, with loss of appetite and loss of weight. The diagnosis is easily made from a simple blood test, and can be confirmed by examination of a small piece of the temporal artery under the microscope (and finding 'giant cells').

Because a major complication is blindness, early diagnosis is important. The headache disappears completely following treatment with steroids, and blindness is prevented.

Brain tumour

Of all the causes of headache, this is the one that is feared most. In fact, it occurs in only a very small minority of people with headache and can often be recognised by its characteristics. It is rare to find a tumour in someone whose headaches have lasted longer than three months, unless they have increased in severity. The headache is made worse by coughing, sneezing or bending down (but this can also occur in benign headaches – see below). The headache may wake the person from sleep and tends to be worse in the morning, when there is often associated nausea or vomiting.

Other ominous symptoms include drowsiness, yawning or hiccup. Further investigation is essential, especially if there are other neurological symptoms such as blurred vision, local numbness or weakness.

Benign headaches

These are common and have no serious significance.

A headache that comes on during sleep in middle-aged or older people, most often women, is called *hypnic headache*. This typically wakes the sufferer in the middle of the night on a regular basis, often several times. It is throbbing in nature and lasts about an hour.

A less common variety that occurs during sleep is the *'exploding' headache*, waking the person with a painful sensation as if an explosion has taken place in the head. Although the sensation soon goes, it leaves the person with a sense of fear, sweating and a rapid pulse rate.

Sleep apnoea is a condition in which there is a temporary stop in breathing during sleep. It may manifest as a morning headache as well as daytime fatigue. If this condition is suspected, investigation in a sleep laboratory is required. If the diagnosis is confirmed, treatment is by means of a machine that produces extra oxygen, keeping the airway open and so getting rid of the cessation in breathing.

Another rare type of benign headache is called *jabs and jolts*, because it feels like a sharp jab with a needle in the corner of the eye. Although it lasts only a matter of seconds, it can recur several times a day. If it happens in someone with migraine, it tends to occur on the same side as the migraine headache. When several attacks come within just a few minutes, they can be quite alarming. Called *idiopathic stabbing pains*, they are benign and not a warning of a more dangerous condition.

Chronic paroxysmal hemicrania is the name for a combination of stabbing pains on one side of the body with drooping of the eyelid on that side, and watering and redness of the eye. The symptoms are like those of cluster headaches but the individual painful attacks are much shorter – seconds or minutes rather than an hour or two. This condition is much more rare and, like cluster headaches, responds to the anti-inflammatory drug indometacin.

Chronic daily headache is a continuous headache that occurs daily for over six months. It was discussed earlier in this chapter.

3
Post-traumatic headache

Post-traumatic headaches occur after trauma to the head or neck, which happens most often in a motor vehicle accident. The impact produces the sudden movement of the person's head forward and then backward, resulting in *flexion–extension* of the neck, giving a *whiplash injury*. If the head also hits some part of the car, there will be varying degrees of head injury. With trauma to the scalp, the nerves under the surface of the skin are damaged and, when healed, may be covered with scar tissue to become the site of continual pain. Where the base of skull adjoins the neck may also be the site of significant pain, with irritation of the occipital nerves which travel from the back to the top of the head. Depending on their symptoms and signs, these headaches may be diagnosed as migraine and/or tension-type headaches.

The nature of the headache determines the treatment:

- People with migraine will be treated with appropriate drugs: preventive (prophylactic) anti-migraine medication or a triptan for attacks.
- Tension-type headache can be treated with tricyclics for prevention and with non-steroidal anti-inflammatory drugs (NSAIDs) for acute attacks.

If there is an aura, nausea and light and sound sensitivity, the headaches are called *post-traumatic migraine*. If none of these symptoms is present but there is a pressure around the head they are called *post-traumatic tension-type headache* (see the discussion of tension-type headache in Chapter 2). Both of these types of headaches can be extremely debilitating and are a major reason why, after such an accident, many people cannot rapidly return to work.

The doctor determines which sort of headache is present and treats it accordingly: post-traumatic migraine as migraine and post-traumatic tension-type headache as tension-type headache. Failure to understand this means that the headaches will be regarded simply as part of the pain in the back or the neck and treated with pain-killers, which can result in prolonging the person's suffering.

The pain at the back of the head may be due to irritation of the greater occipital nerves, which run just under the skin. 'Blocking' these nerves with an injection of local anaesthetic, often combined with a steroid (steroids are anti-inflammatory), is a well-known treatment. Another technique is to investigate the *facet* joints, which are on each vertebra and adjoin (articulate with) each other in the neck (the cervical spine). Injection of local anaesthetic and steroid into these joints – *facet joint block* – is often successful; the injection is done under X-ray control to check that the needle is correctly in the joint. When there is a good response, the nerve roots that supply the facet joints can be permanently interrupted by the operation *facet joint rhizolysis* (*rhizo* is the Greek for 'root').

Although people with post-traumatic headaches improve within six weeks to six months, up to 15 per cent of them may still be suffering ten years after the accident – a significant problem. Some of these accident victims are often treated extremely poorly: their concerns are dismissed and their complaints are treated as lies or malingering, and they may be misunderstood by the insurance industry.

> *William Yates, a 34-year-old international employment lawyer, was involved in a road accident. The taxi in which he was travelling went into a spin, flipped over, crashed into a wall and was a write-off. He hit the right side of the back of his head (the right occipital area). As a result, he developed headaches in that area which then spread to his whole head. He felt sleepy all the time, had no energy and became irritable. His right arm trembled and his memory and concentration were poor. In the middle of an important arbitration, he was worried that he could not concentrate well enough to be effective. He had been on his university's wine-tasting team but now could hardly taste anything.*

Examination revealed mild nystagmus (involuntary rhythmic movement of the eyes) on looking to the left and there was a slight drift downwards of his right arm when he held his arms out in front of him. There was tenderness of his neck and in the right occipital area, with loss of sensation in the distribution of the right occipital nerve. MRI of the brain was negative although it was not done until three months after the accident. Neuropsychological testing revealed a decrease in his performance of rapid alternating movements as well as in attention and memory.

He was treated with physiotherapy for the neck pain. When the headaches had a throbbing or pulsating quality, they responded to a triptan. He was also given amitriptyline as preventive (25mg at night) and naproxen, a pain-killer (500mg twice a day) for the lesser (non-throbbing) headaches. Five months after the taxi accident, another car in which he was travelling was 'rear-ended', as a result of which he suffered a whiplash injury in his neck. After this his headaches became worse and he developed dizziness. When seen in follow-up 18 months later, he still had almost daily headaches but they were not severe. He was still somewhat forgetful, and still could not smell truffles.

This case is a typical example of post-traumatic syndrome in which headache is the most common symptom after a whiplash injury. There may be many other symptoms, including dizziness, mood changes, and intellectual and sleep disturbances. They may occur even if there was no loss of consciousness. There may be true giddiness (vertigo) made worse by changing position, or the giddiness may be ill-defined and felt just as unsteadiness.

The mechanisms of post-traumatic headache

Specific damage to the structures in the neck can give rise to neck pain, leading to pain in the head and sometimes producing a true migraine attack. People who have never suffered from migraine before can develop this after even a minor head or neck injury.

Predisposing conditions

Pre-existing headache may be a risk factor in the development of post-traumatic headache, as may a history of neck pain. People who have had migraine can develop more frequent or more severe attacks.

The nature of the headache

Migraine with aura and cluster headaches can also occur after trauma. It is estimated that about one-quarter of people with head injury will still have headaches six months after the incident. Chronic headache after trauma can be produced by overuse of pain-killers in the same manner as medication-overuse headache.

Examination of the person with post-traumatic headache

A doctor investigating the possibility of post-traumatic headache needs to know whether there was loss of consciousness, the duration of any loss of memory for the time before and after the accident and whether there was any skull or neck fracture. Previous headache history is necessary as well as any other relevant details about past illness, personality and occupation. The physical examination should focus on the presence of tender areas in the head and neck and the mobility of the neck, as well as the general and neurological assessments. Any effects on sleep and mood also need to be evaluated.

Investigation of the person with post-traumatic headache

This will include scanning of the brain using: computed tomography (CT), which involves X-rays; magnetic resonance imaging (MRI), which does not involve X-rays; or, less frequently, single photon emission computed tomography (SPECT), which involves the use of radioactive isotopes. When there is a possibility of epilepsy as well as the headaches, electroencephalography (EEG) is indicated.

Most patients with mild or moderate head injury have some abnormalities visible on MRI immediately after the trauma but these largely resolve within one month. Problems in attention and concentration usually resolve within six weeks of the injury, and other psychological symptoms within about three months.

Dysfunction of the temporo-mandibular joint

The temporo-mandibular joint is just in front of the ear, between the lower jaw (mandible) and the lower part of the temporal bone of the skull. Dysfunction of this joint is common after trauma, and dental assessment may be necessary. An MRI of the joints may be necessary; treatment may involve surgery.

Cervical headache

Pain in the neck is extremely common after road traffic accidents, and may give rise to post-traumatic headaches. Nerve blocks can be efficacious but of more value are 'diagnostic facet joint blocks', which are performed under X-ray control. If the blocks are positive, facet joint rhizolysis (explained earlier) can provide sustained relief. The relief obtained can last up to six months and sometimes longer. Injection of botulinum toxin into the neck can lessen the painful spasm, increase range of movement and improve the headache; it has been useful in both migraine and tension-type headache. (Botulinum is discussed in Chapter 9.)

There is some evidence for the effectiveness of physiotherapy, acupuncture and chiropractic treatment. Some health professionals are sufficiently convinced of their efficacy in certain cases that the treatments are available through the NHS in some areas.

The long-term outlook

Many people still have post-traumatic headaches one month after their injury. The number diminishes gradually but about one-fifth may still be experiencing these headaches four years later. Other symptoms of the post-traumatic syndrome may persist for many years.

4
Who gets migraine?

Nearly everyone has a headache at some time in their lives but migraine with its special features affects only a minority. Based on the International Headache Society's criteria for the diagnosis of the condition, migraine affects 5 per cent of men and 17 per cent of women at some stage in their lives. This, however, is a strict definition that was introduced for the primary purpose of research, both for treatment and for genetic studies; the true number of people affected is probably double these figures – a very large segment of the population. The reason why it is more common in women is not precisely known but this sex difference could be a clue as to one of its causes.

Migraine affects at least 6 million people in the UK – more than those with diabetes, asthma and epilepsy combined. It is responsible for the loss of over 18 million working days each year and costs the economy around £1 billion in lost production because of the time taken off work, the cost of replacement staff and periods when employees are working under par during attacks.

That figure is an under-estimate, as the calculation is based on health certificates, which are issued only for three or more days off work, and most people with migraine are often away for less than this during any one attack. (A survey done in the 1970s revealed that 21 per cent of Members of Parliament had migraine and that each one lost an average of four work-days a year.) Those who persist in working during an attack are likely to be less efficient, which also contributes to the problems caused by migraine. Questionnaires designed to evaluate the disability caused by migraine have shown that people with migraine perceive themselves to be as disabled as those suffering from diabetes or angina.

The age at which migraine begins varies. It usually starts in adolescence and young adulthood but there will often have been warnings in childhood of its likely development.

Migraine in children

Studies of children have found that slightly more boys than girls have migraine. After puberty, however, the ratio changes and by the late teens or early twenties the proportion of female to male reaches the adult figure of 3:1. Children often have a condition called *migraine equivalents*, which usually take the form of periodic (cyclical) vomiting not due to any obvious cause such as over-indulgence of food. These 'bilious attacks' can occur once a month but last no more than a day (see also 'Abdominal migraine' in Chapter 1).

Recurrent abdominal pain with or without vomiting is another warning that the child may develop migrainous headaches in later years. Children who are prone to travel sickness are another group with a tendency to develop migraine in later life.

In all these cases, a clue as to the true nature of the condition will often be found in the family because there is very likely to be a close relative with migrainous headaches.

Migraine in older people

Older people do not have migraine as commonly or as severely as the young. There are, however, exceptions to this rule. Many women whose migraine is worse at the time of their menstrual period are told that their attacks will disappear with the menopause. This is sometimes, but not always, the case. Indeed, in some women, the headaches can be worse at the menopause.

There is little doubt, though, that attacks change their characteristics during life. For example, headache and vomiting become less severe and in many cases the disorder becomes less troublesome. Acephalgic migraine (see the case history of Charles Dodds in Chapter 1) is common in older people. Those who have migraine with aura may lose the headache and nausea but continue with attacks of visual aura without any other symptoms.

Heredity

Migraine is a familial disorder – it tends to run in the family. Indeed, a family history of migraine is further evidence that a headache sufferer has migraine. Estimates of how frequently it runs in families will depend on how widely the term 'family' is extended. If the family history is taken just from the individual with migraine, about 50 per cent will know of an affected relative; however, if close (first-degree) relatives such as parents, siblings and children are questioned, the figure rises to 90 per cent.

The precise way in which migraine is inherited is not as simple as, for example, the inheritance of blood groups. In fact, it is not scientifically accurate to say that headaches are 'inherited' – only the *tendency* to have certain types of headaches. There are rare types in which the genetics have been worked out and even the precise chromosome on which the gene is located. One of them is *familial hemiplegic migraine*, which is associated with paralysis of one half of the body during attacks; the relevant gene is located on chromosome 19. The abnormality is on the cell membrane, which governs the passage of chemicals passing into and out of the cell. When the relevant gene is present on chromosome 19, the passage of calcium through the membrane is abnormal, which then alters the conductivity of the nerve cell to predispose to a migraine attack.

The migrainous personality

From the eighteenth century until relatively recently, it was thought that people in the upper strata of society suffered more from migraine. Scientific studies have shown, however, that migraine attacks occur in all social classes, irrespective of intelligence or income. The reason why the myth persisted for two centuries is that only the better-off people could have afforded doctors' fees. Even today, only a minority of people with migraine go to their doctor about their condition.

Another myth was that hard-working, conscientious perfectionists were more likely to have migraine, a subjective view that migrainous doctors might have found it hard to dispute! Objective studies confirm that no one type of personality is more prone than others; in fact, migraine occurs just as frequently in people who are neither obsessional nor compulsive. Although some people with migraine are aggressive, demanding and distrustful, these traits are no more common than in the general population. Such characteristics may be the result of repeated headaches rather than the cause of migraine.

There is little doubt that stress of different kinds can predispose to migraine attacks, and this is discussed more fully in later chapters.

Weekend migraine

Although migraine is often thought of as a stress disease, many people get attacks only when they are relaxing at weekends or on holiday; this may be due to changes in habits such as sleeping longer or a change in coffee intake. People prone to weekend migraine may drink more coffee and tea during the week; at the weekend, they drink less coffee and tea, and so the migraine may be due to caffeine withdrawal. Another explanation is that they do not have to get up early, and it is the change in sleep pattern that triggers an attack. For this reason some people with migraine try to get up at the same time on weekends as they do during the week. Also implicated as a possible trigger is a change in eating pattern.

Others will get attacks only when they are anticipating an exciting event, such as a party; this can be so distinctive that they refuse social invitations in the certain knowledge that acceptance will provoke an attack.

Relation of migraine to other disorders

Although there are many conditions that are claimed to produce pain in the head region (e.g. sinusitis, high blood pressure, eye strain), there is no proof that these conditions predispose to migraine. Nevertheless, treatment of high blood pressure often lessens the frequency of migraine attacks.

There are conditions that have a 'co-morbidity' with migraine. This means that, statistically, they are found more often in people with migraine but it does not mean that the conditions necessarily have a common cause. For example, anxiety, depression, panic attacks and stroke are co-morbid with migraine. The risk of stroke in people with migraine, especially young women who smoke, use the contraceptive pill and who have migraine with aura, is four times higher than that of 'controls' – people from the general population – but the risk is still extremely small.

Many people with migraine notice that their attacks are more frequent when they are 'run-down' or suffering from general upsets. For example, Charles Dodds (mentioned in Chapter 1), on returning from a lecture tour in India, suddenly developed frequent (sometimes twice-daily) attacks of migraine, which were produced by slight stress, such as a short walk. A blood test revealed evidence of an infection, which later proved to be an inflammatory bowel disorder. When that condition was cured with treatment, Charles had no further migraine attacks.

5
Why does the head ache?

Because almost everyone suffers from headache at some time, it is often not regarded as a disease. Nevertheless, it is a disease (in the sense of not being at ease): headache can interfere considerably with the lives of significant numbers of people, so it is illogical to regard it as a normal occurrence. Because the changes occurring in the body are subtle, it is exceedingly difficult to analyse those taking place during headaches, even with sophisticated research tools. Often, any abnormality discovered is then found to be only secondary to pain, or not to be present in all those with the same symptoms. By comparison, the understanding of an obvious abnormality such as a chest infection is simple – not only can changes be seen on an X-ray but also the germ that has caused the infection can be grown in the laboratory.

The fact that a number of people have a specific form of headache does not necessarily mean that the cause is the same in all of them. In the same way, a blocked nose and sore throat may be caused by infection with germs or by allergy; the symptoms can be identical but the treatment of each is very different: for example, treating a 'runny' nose due to hay-fever or a virus with antibiotics is worse than useless.

The situation in distinguishing between headaches is comparable, except that a good deal is known about the structures concerned with pain and the nerves that carry that sensation.

The pathway of pain

There are pathways in the nervous system that help us appreciate our environment, whether by sight, touch or hearing. Each sense organ can be regarded as an extension, or the sensitive area, of a nerve that is linked to the brain. In the eyes, the light-sensitive cells in the back of the eyeball (retina) are linked together in specific patterns that are then transmitted by the optic nerves to a 'relay station' at the back of the brain. In lower animals, much organisation of incoming information is carried out here, but in humans and other primates most of the processing occurs in the grey matter of the brain, the cortex, where the cell bodies of the neurones are. Here, the shape

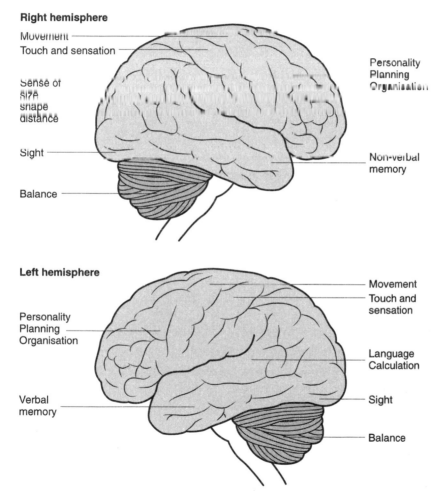

Right hemisphere

Movement
Touch and sensation

Sense of
size
shape
distance

Sight

Balance

Personality
Planning
Organisation

Non-verbal
memory

Left hemisphere

Personality
Planning
Organisation

Verbal
memory

Movement
Touch and
sensation

Language
Calculation

Sight

Balance

Figure 5.1 Some of the various functions controlled by different parts of the brain.

perceived is compared with stored information and recognition occurs when the pattern is matched with memory. A label is supplied by an area of the brain concerned with memory and we now have a conscious appreciation of what the object is. A similar process occurs with the recognition of sounds but, in this case, different areas of the brain are involved. Figure 5.1 shows which parts of the brain control the various functions.

Touch (tactile sensation) is different from seeing and hearing in that the impulses have to travel a greater distance up the spinal cord to the brain, except in the case of sensation from the face. The other varieties of sensation include temperature, superficial pain and deep pain. Impulses travel along nerve fibres from sensitive structures in the skin to the spinal cord where they pass their messages on to nerve tracts – long nerve fibres that are grouped together. These fibres travel to the brain where two things happen. The first is that the location of the sensation is pinpointed to a specific part of the brain, which is specifically activated; the second event is a general alerting reaction so that other areas of the brain go into a state of expectancy. Because of this activation (which can be measured electrically) there is an increased flow of blood to the nerve cells. Complex patterns of skin stimulation can be analysed by the brain in much the same way as patterns of light and sound are perceived by our eyes and ears.

The structures in the skin or other tissues that receive painful stimuli are a specific type, and are different from those sensitive to touch and temperature. Pain sensation is served by two types of nerve fibre, fast and slow, each of which transmits pain of a different character: the fast fibre transmits discrete, sharp pain whilst the slow fibre produces dull and diffuse pain. Slow-conducting fibres also transmit the sensation of itch; this is why scratching helps – it blocks the itch sensation by pain. This idea of blocking pain by stimulating certain nerves may explain why acupuncture and electrical stimulation work (see Chapter 8).

Referred pain

The place where the pain seems to be is not necessarily where the cause lies: the pain can be felt in some other part of the body – *referred pain*. The explanation for this lies in the fact that the two areas are supplied by the same nerve; for example, someone with an inflamed gall bladder may feel pain in the right shoulder, as the nerve supply to both the gall bladder and the right shoulder is the same. A similar problem may arise when a person has a pain at the lower end of the gullet, which may be indistinguishable from pain arising in the heart.

The response to pain

Whatever the cause of the stimulus, sudden pain has three effects:

- It triggers an early avoidance response by reflexes controlled in the spinal cord (e.g. we take our hand out of the fire before we even feel the pain).
- Next, the impulse travels to the brain, where it activates a particular area that locates and assesses the pain.
- Then the whole brain is activated and thrown into a state of readiness.

Chronic (long-standing) pain differs from acute (short-term) pain in that the avoidance response does not occur. The specific response to feeling, or appreciating, pain still takes place but the activation of the brain is variable, possibly because the persistent stress of chronic pain produces chemical changes in the body that cause lack of concentration, depression and anxiety. In some people, areas of the brain dealing with emotions become activated, causing a change in behaviour. With treatment, these areas return to normal.

In appreciating pain, another important factor is attention. A toothache is often worse at night on going to bed but, as soon as the mind is occupied and engrossed, the pain subsides into the background. (This aspect is used in certain forms of meditation and in hypnosis, where the conscious mind can be distracted or 'shut out' entirely.) This factor is important, because the appreciation of chronic pain varies not only from one person to another but also in the same individual, depending on his or her state of mind. People who are depressed, whether because of the chronic recurrent pain or for other reasons, are less likely to put up resistance to the continuous attack on their pain sense.

The pain threshold

We all have different responses to pain, not only in our conscious reaction but also in the amount of pain required to impinge on our consciousness. This pain threshold can easily be tested by, for instance, asking someone when a certain temperature applied to their skin becomes painful. In one such experiment a 100-watt lamp was focused on a subject's blackened forehead for three seconds; the intensity of the lamp could be varied, and the lowest level of illumination producing minimal pain (a prickling sensation on the forehead) was taken as the pain threshold. There was remarkable similarity in this value as long as the subjects concentrated on the task in hand. Distraction, suggestion and hypnosis could raise this threshold by 35 per cent, as could pain-killers. Pain thresholds vary greatly and become unpredictable in people who are tired or anxious. Scientific, objective methods of measurement and analysis are very necessary in the study of what is, in the final analysis, a subjective complaint.

People tend to suppress the memory of unpleasant events, so it is often difficult to give an accurate account of previous pain. The suppression is partly due to unconscious forgetting, and possibly also because the chemicals produced by the pain dull the memory.

Response to pain also depends to some extent on sociological factors. People in social classes 1 and 2 are more likely to complain of headache, a tendency that has given the false impression that they are more prone to get headaches. In fact, given equal access to healthcare, all strata of society are affected equally.

The brain itself is insensitive to pain – neurosurgeons can operate on it without general anaesthesia. The structures in the head that feel pain are the blood vessels and the coverings of the brain (the meninges). The pain felt in migrainous headaches is conveyed by the trigemino-vascular system (see 'Innervation of the blood vessels', later): the pressure of swollen blood vessels against the sensitive membranes that line the skull.

The coverings of the brain

The brain is enveloped by three coverings, or meninges (see Figure 5.2). The dura mater is the outer covering attached to the

Inside of the skull where, in certain places, it makes reinforcing sheets.

Underlying the dura mater is the arachnoid mater, which is closely opposed to another very fine layer that closely surrounds the brain and its blood vessels – the pia mater. Between the arachnoid mater and the pia mater is a fluid that bathes and protects the brain and spinal cord – the cerebrospinal fluid.

The skull itself has a covering (the periosteum), which contains short blood vessels. The bone of the skull is insensitive to pain but the periosteum has pain receptors and is very sensitive, particularly in areas over the brow, the temples and at the back of the head; stretching of the periosteum, caused by inflammation or growths, will cause severe pain. Although the brain itself does not feel pain, all the main arteries supplying the dura mater and some of the smaller branches are sensitive, as are the blood vessels of the scalp, so the stretching of an artery on one side will cause severe pain on that side.

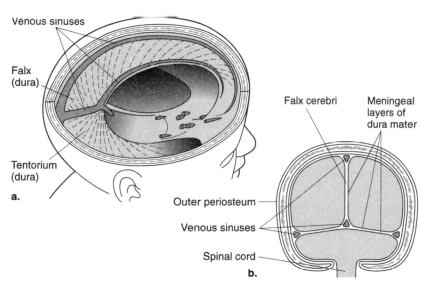

Figure 5.2 Pain-sensitive structures in the skull. In this diagram the brain has been removed, showing the pain-sensitive supporting structures. The venous sinuses lie in the dura mater, which stretches down the centre of the skull (the falx) and horizontally across the back of the skull (the tentorium). The periosteum covers both sides of the skull bones; the inner layer adheres to the dura mater; the pia and arachnoid are stuck together, covering the brain, but separate below where the spinal cord ends.

The dura above the tentorium, which divides the front (the cerebral hemispheres) and back of the brain (the cerebellum), is entirely insensitive to pain, except near the venous sinuses and areas of the main arteries. The dura covering the floor of the skull in the front area is very sensitive and the pain produced spreads to behind the eye. The dura lining the back of the brain is equally sensitive but not that covering the floor of the areas below the temporal lobes (see Chapter 1). The falx is insensitive to pain in its front part except for where it connects with the area above the nose.

Pressure on the tentorium produces pain in the area around the forehead, eye and ear on the same side. The great venous sinuses are very sensitive to pain but the smaller sinuses less so; stimulation of the smaller sinuses at the back of the head causes pain over the forehead and eye.

The smaller arteries of the brain, as opposed to the main blood vessels, are insensitive to pain. The pain caused by widening (dilation) of the internal carotid artery inside the skull is dull, throbbing and eventually nauseating; it is localised behind the eye and over the temple on the same side as the stimulus.

Pain is caused by both distension and diminution in size of the brain's ventricles – the normal cavities of the brain that produce and contain the cerebrospinal fluid (CSF) surrounding and circulating around the brain and spinal cord. A headache usually occurs after a spinal tap (lumbar puncture), when CSF is removed for analysis. This headache is due to low CSF pressure caused by the removal of CSF during the procedure and subsequent leaking through the hole made in the dura; this is why rest in bed is always required afterwards.

The cranial nerves

There are twelve pairs of cranial nerves – the nerves that arise from the brain itself – but all the pain impulses in the head are carried by only two of them, the fifth and ninth cranial nerves, which also serve most of the other sensations felt in the head and face. Pain can also be produced by stimulating the tenth and eleventh cranial nerves, as well as nerves coming from the spinal cord in the upper part of the neck; this pain is felt at the back and top of the head.

The fifth cranial, or trigeminal, nerve arises from an area in the upper part of the hind-brain where its control centre (nucleus) lies and extends deep in the spinal cord of the neck. In this part of the nucleus the areas of the face are represented in a concentric way like the layers of an onion, so damage to the upper part can cause tingling or loss of sensation round the lips. The main trunk of the trigeminal nerve splits into three branches in an area of the skull near to the front of the upper part of the jaw bone: the upper branch goes to the area of face above the eye and forehead, the middle branch to the cheek and the lower branch to the lower jaw. There is, of course, an identical nerve on the other side of the face. When a dentist anaesthetises part of the jaw, it is a branch of this nerve that is being blocked.

Much of the knowledge regarding these pain pathways was obtained from experiments on volunteers undergoing operations; this speaks volumes for the co-operation and interest of the volunteers! The methods employed in these experiments varied – e.g. mild electric shocks and traction – but they were not the sort of stimuli that cause headaches in everyday life.

The autonomic nervous system

The walls of the blood vessels consist of three layers: an outer and an inner layer, and a middle layer that is muscle. The muscle 'coats' are supplied by nerves but, unlike the nerves relaying pain sensations, their functions are similar to those of nerves going to other muscle fibres: stimulation causes the muscle to contract and so narrows the blood vessels.

These nerves come from part of the nervous system that, because it deals with functions not usually under control of the conscious mind, is called the autonomic nervous system. This system is in two parts – the sympathetic and the parasympathetic – each of which has different actions.

The sympathetic nervous system increases tension (tone) of the blood vessel walls, making them more resistant to increases in blood pressure; it also has effects on the heart, speeding its action, as well as on the circulation to other organs. It is the sympathetic system that takes over in situations of danger in the well-known 'fight or flight' situation. Activation of this system causes release of adrenaline from the adrenal gland, which makes us ready for action – for example, the pupils of our eyes are widened. Stimulating the sympathetic system decreases the blood vessel calibre, so decreasing blood flow to the skin. This can be increased by such techniques as putting the hands in hot water, relaxation or taking nitroglycerine (a drug used to treat angina because it dilates blood vessels and lowers blood pressure, thereby lessening the strain on the heart).

The parasympathetic system has opposite actions. For example, when the relevant nerves are stimulated, the pupils of the eyes will narrow. It slows the heart and causes a general relaxation of the blood vessels.

Other factors that control blood vessel diameter are (in the area of the blood vessels) changes in the concentration of carbon dioxide and acidity of the blood, increases of which will cause the blood vessels to dilate. These are not the sort of stimuli that cause headaches in everyday life. More recently pain has been induced in volunteers by injecting their foreheads with a chilli-like compound called capsaicin. This extremely irritative substance causes intense pain in areas where the headaches usually occur. Using this substance it is possible to determine which part of the brain responds to the pain produced in a particular area of the body. This mechanism is quite separate from the spontaneous activity of the brain; an alteration in this activity may be the direct cause of the pain initially.

The pain in headache is due to inflammation and dilation of the blood vessels. The blood vessels become inflamed because of substances released by the nerves around them. As the inflamed blood vessels dilate, each pulse beat produces a throbbing pain. Before the headache phase of migraine with aura there is a wave of electrical activity that spreads across the brain (called spreading depression), bringing with it a line of increased blood flow followed by diminished blood flow. Although this is still not fully understood, it seems to be a response of certain brains to stimulation – either external or internal. The spread of activation followed by diminished blood flow may account for some of the neurological features that occur during an attack. The most common pattern is a visual disturbance (i.e. an aura, as discussed in Chapter 1) but this can be accompanied by abnormalities of sensation in the arms, legs or face as well as difficulties with thought, memory and speech.

The blood vessels and the brain

The brain is enclosed in a container of bone (the skull) which in turn is covered by a fibrous structure and skin (the scalp). The scalp is attached by muscles to the forehead and to the bones of the neck, so tensing these muscles causes stretching of the scalp. Beneath the skin there are numerous blood vessels – arteries taking blood from the heart and veins returning blood to it. The scalp arteries arise from the large carotid artery, which divides in the neck into two branches (see Figure 5.3). One of these, the external carotid artery, sends blood to the outside of the skull and to the coverings of the brain in the skull, while the other branch, the internal carotid artery, enters the skull to join with vessels originating from the vertebral artery. The blood supply to the brain is from branches of the left and right internal carotid arteries which, with the vertebral arteries, form a communication round the base of the brain – the circle of Willis (Figure 5.4). From this 'circle', branches go to the front, centre and back of the

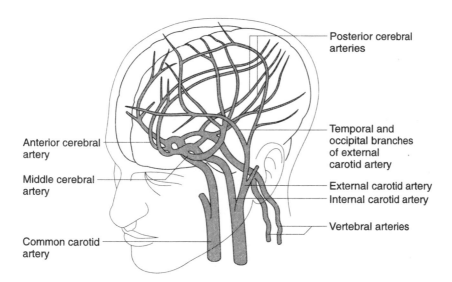

Figure 5.3 The distribution of arteries inside and outside the skull. The internal carotid artery divides to form the anterior and middle cerebral arteries. The two vertebral arteries join to form the basilar artery, which divides into the posterior cerebral arteries. The external carotid artery gives rise to numerous branches outside the skull, including the temporal and occipital arteries.

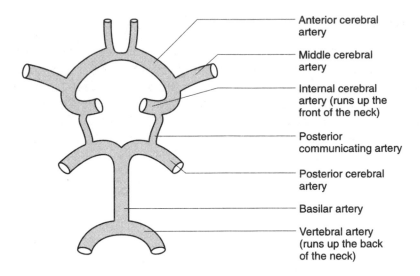

Figure 5.4 The blood supply to the brain, including the 'circle of Willis'

brain, sending out a network of ever-finer vessels that dive deep into the substance of the brain.

Veins drain the blood from the brain and channel it into a series of large veins (venous sinuses) closely attached to the brain coverings. From these, the blood travels either by way of the jugular veins or by communications through the skull, to join with blood draining from the scalp and returning eventually to the heart.

The blood supply

The sites in the head that give rise to pain are related to blood vessels, and the relation between these and the structures they supply are of paramount importance (see Figures 5.2–5.4).

Blood vessels, especially arteries, have a muscular coat that enables them to change their diameter. These changes alter the amount of, as well as the resistance to, blood flow. The smallest blood vessels – the capillaries – form a network to supply organs with oxygen and nutrients, without which body tissues die. Blood flow is regulated by demands of the tissues, the nervous system controlling the opening or closing of parts of the capillary system.

Cerebral blood flow

Exciting scientific discoveries in the 1970s revolutionised our ideas of the relation between thought and blood flow. Previously it had been considered that thinking did not use any significant amount of energy and that blood flow to the brain was constant. It is now known, however, that when groups of brain cells are activated they use up oxygen, produce carbon dioxide and cause an increase in blood flow to that area by dilating the blood vessels.

Early research revealed that these changes could be followed using radioactive tracers injected into the arteries, and remarkable pictures were obtained. For instance, the pattern of blood flow in someone at rest is markedly increased in the frontal areas of the brain; if the person is talking, there is a decrease of flow to these areas while part of the temporal lobe shows a marked increase of activity – confirmation of the long-held theory that this area is a centre for language. Similar things happen when other intellectual activities are undertaken, so these research techniques show which particular area of the brain exercises certain functions.

Pain increases the metabolism in the brain and so dilates its blood vessels. This increase in vessel diameter makes it more difficult for the body to control local changes to blood flow, which could explain why thinking becomes more difficult during severe pain. A paradox is that pain, like stress, increases activity in the sympathetic nervous system yet it increases blood flow to the brain; the resulting vasoconstriction would be expected to decrease it. The answer is probably that the sympathetic nervous system controls the larger, so-called resistance, vessels, whereas pain in this context activates local capillaries.

The system that controls blood flow to the brain is highly complex, as it is affected by nervous factors, chemicals (amines) circulating in the body and outside factors such as pain, as well as by our mental processes. The importance of the last factor was highlighted by asking volunteers to solve problems of mental arithmetic while their brain blood flow was being measured. There was a slight increase to appropriate areas but this became greatly magnified when they were offered money for the successful solution to the problems! This indicates that motivation and concentration have a direct effect on the flow of blood to the brain.

Innervation of the blood vessels

The nerves to the blood vessels in the linings of the brain (the meninges) and the larger blood vessels going to the brain are different. The fifth cranial nerve, the trigeminal, is the main one, and the trigemino-vascular system functions as a unit. An area in the brain stem, at the back of the brain, becomes active and causes a 'firing' of the fifth nerve back along its sensory fibres, causing the release of substances that, in turn, cause inflammation around the blood vessels. These substances are varied but include substance P and calcitonin and gene-related peptide, which are known to cause inflammation in experimental situations. Why the 'generator' in the brain stem acts in this way is not known but there are a number of triggers (discussed in Chapter 6).

One of the most important factors is genetic. Over 90 per cent of people with migraine have a relative with migraine. This suggests that those with migraine have inherited an abnormal mechanism releasing certain chemical substances, which can act on the trigemino-vascular system, to cause headache and the other features of migraine. One system that has been identified is the calcium channel. In people whose headaches are accompanied by paralysis of one side of the body (*familial hemiplegic migraine*, discussed in Chapter 1), 'information' that affects this channel is carried on chromosome 19. This relates to migraine in that the calcium channels affect the activity of the nerves and blood vessels.

Other conditions have been implicated in intermittent abnormalities of certain proteins that control the flow of ions through cell membranes. One is the disease *episodic ataxia* in which, from time to time, affected people become unsteady and their speech is slurred, making it seem as though they are drunk. This condition lasts between several hours and days. Another condition that is thought to be an abnormality of ionic channels is *periodic paralysis*. Found especially in certain ethnic groups (e.g. people from the Philippines), it causes paralysis from time to time. Understanding of these so-called channelopathies may explain a variety of disorders in which changes are episodic rather than constant.

6
What brings on a migraine attack?

Much is known about the factors that make blood vessels change their size but it is still uncertain what triggers a migraine attack. Although only a minority of people have migraine, it is possible that others would as well in certain circumstances. Even those with migraine vary enormously in their susceptibility to attacks – from those who have almost continual attacks to others who get them only once in many years.

Just as there are many factors in the tendency to migraine (e.g. age, sex, family history), so there are even more that can (or are said to) trigger an attack. The list of these 'provocative' factors is large and includes:

dietary

irregular meals

fasting

change in caffeine intake

alcohol

food additives such as monosodium glutamate and, anecdotally, aspartame

certain foods: cured meats, cheese, chocolate, citrus fruits, fried foods, butter

physical

hard work

exercise

sexual intercourse

hormonal

menstruation

oral contraceptives

menopause

biological

changes in biological rhythm

changes in sleep pattern

high blood pressure
   (hypertension)

psychological

anxiety

tension

depression

shock

frustration

anecdotal

strong smells (e.g. perfume,
   paint, flowers)

glare, bright/flickering lights

weather/environment changes

cold

hot baths, saunas

loud noise

other facial pains (e.g. toothache)

head colds

hay-fever

poor posture

smoking

Although the number here seems large, it is not comprehensive – hence the claim that 'almost anything' can spark off a migraine attack. For this reason, many people with migraine find it difficult to pinpoint the actual trigger. More often than not, the trigger is a combination of more than one factor, of which stress is the most common. For these reasons, a migraine specialist will ask a patient to keep a headache or migraine diary in which such aspects as food, pattern of meals, fluid intake, menstruation, and so on are recorded along with the attacks.

Stress

'Stress' is one of the most misused words in the English language, and its precise meaning is often forgotten. It is defined in the *Shorter Oxford Dictionary* as a 'demand upon energy'. This is a difficult concept to apply to the human body and not a factor that can easily be measured. Although breaking a leg is caused by undue stress, it is not this mechanical use of the word that is usually intended; more often, the implication is a mental strain with a consequent decreased ability to cope. For some people stress is a welcome challenge to be overcome and they are unhappy without some tension in their lives; others cannot tolerate any form of stress. Most people fall between these two extremes, their responses depending on the situation.

Many studies have been made of stress, particularly in its relation to heart disease. Based on these studies people have been classified into two groups: type A and type B. The A type takes stress badly, becoming tense, edgy and 'rushing about'; the B type is more relaxed and, when under stress, tends to use the situation in a constructive manner. Someone who is type A is almost twice as likely to develop heart attacks as a type B person. Comparable studies have not yet been done in relation to migraine but personality may play a part in determining who gets migraine, as the different responses to stress are important in determining the frequency of attacks.

It is likely that stress is related to biochemical changes in the body but not necessarily the increased production of adrenaline or noradrenaline.

Dietary factors

Fasting

It is well known that going without food can bring on an attack of migraine. The explanation often given is that, during fasting, the sugar in the blood falls to a low level (hypoglycaemia) and this provokes an attack. In fact, there are normally body reserves that can be converted to glucose during fasting so that the blood sugar level does not become abnormally low.

When sugar is eaten, the hormone insulin is released. The action of insulin is to lower the blood sugar level, and it does this in everyone, but the low levels may last longer than expected in people who get migraine. Sugar is absorbed in the same way by everyone but the release of insulin in response might not be quite the same in people with migraine. A study using a hormone that releases glucose (glucagon) revealed that there was a consistently smaller resultant rise of blood glucose in people with migraine, and that other abnormalities also took longer to return to normal. However, these findings have not been fully confirmed. There is no scientific evidence that people with a migraine attack have a lower level of blood sugar than have others. It is probable that other changes, such as the release of free fatty acids in the blood associated with fasting, are the trigger factors.

Food headaches

We saw in Chapter 2 that there are chemical substances in certain foods that can cause a headache – for example the 'Chinese restaurant' syndrome (monosodium glutamate), the hot-dog headache (nitrites), and other foods that produce headache because of their physical characteristics (e.g. ice-cream headache). These headaches are not usually typically migrainous. Probably less than 10 per cent of migraine attacks are due to food alone, not least because other trigger factors (e.g. tiredness or menstruation) are also present.

Cheese
There are some people who get a headache after eating cheese but it is not always the case, as revealed by 'food challenges' – that is, testing whether the food blamed produces an attack; such food challenges usually have a negative result, not producing an attack. The substance that was once thought to be responsible for 'cheese headache' was tyramine, but giving this to cheese-reactive people did not often produce a migraine attack.

Chocolate
This is another substance that has been claimed to provoke migraine. Although chocolate also contains tyramine, it is now claimed that another amine, phenylethylamine, may be responsible. Again, this has not been confirmed by food challenges; phenylethylamine is theoretically more likely to *prevent* migraine because some people who are about to have a headache crave chocolate in order to stave off an attack, which is then blamed on the chocolate.

An experiment was performed with four migrainous people who thought that their attacks were brought on by chocolate. Each week they took a capsule and for four months recorded their headaches. All the capsules looked alike but some contained chocolate whereas the others contained just lactose. The 'guinea-pigs', who happened to be doctors, did not know which capsule was which. At the end of four months, the number of headaches following each type of capsule was found to be the same. This shows how cautious we must be when apportioning blame to trigger factors!

Tea and coffee

The active constituents of tea and coffee include caffeine and theophylline, substances that prevent the breakdown of a high-energy compound, cyclic AMP. The build-up of this substance makes the body far more sensitive to the action of the sympathetic nervous system (discussed in Chapter 5). Caffeine and theophylline have been used in the treatment of headaches, and many drugs given for headache contain caffeine. In some people who have weekend headaches their attack may be caused by taking less caffeine than they do during the week – they are getting a caffeine-withdrawal headache. It is also known that excessive amounts of caffeine can cause headaches.

> *Geoff Hardy had repeated severe attacks of migraine that resisted all forms of treatment. He was found to be highly sensitive to tea and his migraines improved when this was excluded from his diet.*

> *Ida Jones used to get unexplained severe pains and had been labelled as neurotic. But when given tea or coffee by a nasogastric tube (through the nose into the stomach) – so that she could not taste it – she developed the pains and her pulse rate doubled, whereas when she was given water through the tube there was no such effect. After stopping taking tea or coffee, she had no further attacks.*

Alcohol

This is the most common 'food additive' taken, and is known to dilate blood vessels. The 'hangover' headache following excessive alcohol is well known, but this is probably due partly to dehydration (alcohol is a diuretic). Some migraine sufferers are particularly sensitive to alcohol, especially red wine and port. This is not due to the alcohol, as vodka will not give them a migraine attack; it is related to other substances (higher esters, flavonoid phenols) that are present in the drink.

Smoking

Although there is no clear correlation between smoking and migraine, there is no doubt that this habit produces vascular changes; for example, the pulse rate increases after smoking. There is anecdotal evidence that some people with migraine improve after giving up the habit.

Other foods

As well as the foods already mentioned, many others have been said to cause migraine, the more common examples being citrus fruits and meat.

> *Kenneth Lloyd always had an attack some hours after eating pork, but only when tired or under emotional stress. He could eat pork with impunity if he was in 'good condition'. Skin testing (which is not always accurate) determined that he was sensitive not only to pork but also to many other types of food.*

This last case study illustrates the fact that it is not necessarily a single factor that induces an attack. In addition to Kenneth having the propensity to develop the attack, a single stimulus – in this case, pork – might not be enough but another – in this case, fatigue – had to be present as well.

Food allergy

'Allergy' is a vague term but, when used in its medical sense, means an abnormal reaction of the body's immune system to a stimulus in its environment. Because so many disorders are said to be allergic in origin, scientists are reluctant to accept this explanation unless confirmation is obtained by immunological tests. The problem with so-called food allergies causing headache is that it is not really certain what actually causes the symptoms, which may be due to a sensitivity rather than an allergy. When food is digested, many different molecules are released and only one of these could be the culprit. Migraine produced by food is probably due to a sensitivity, rather than to an allergy.

Because food triggers are generally viewed as being associated with a person's sensitivity (not an allergy), doing skin tests on people with migraine to determine what they are allergic to will be of little value. The blood tests depend on the person's serum reacting against certain food molecules and these are not reliable. The only way to find which food produces a migraine is to do 'blind' testing using a nasogastric tube (as with Ida, mentioned above).

Another method is an exclusion diet. The individual eats nothing but one particular food for a month and then every month afterwards adds another food to the combination; if an attack is triggered, the offending food is dropped and another one substituted. This type of testing diet is extremely difficult and tedious, and most people find it impossible to comply with it. However, this approach can sometimes reduce the frequency of headaches.

Physical factors

Exercise can provoke attacks of migraine but regular exercise can prevent them. Exercise is a particular form of stress, with chemical changes taking place – for example, an outpouring of adrenal hormones. This makes the heart beat faster to supply more blood to the exercising muscles, but the excess hormones released are quickly used up.

Hormones

Menstrual migraine

Many women with migraine often relate their attacks to the menstrual cycle. If the week before is considered premenstrual and the week after postmenstrual, three of the four weeks of the cycle could be thought of as closely related to menstruation; it is not surprising, therefore, that most attacks have been associated with menstruation. The action of female hormones (oestrogen and progesterone) on blood vessels in the lining of the womb (the uterus) during the menstrual cycle is of relevance to migraine. The uterine blood vessels become elongated, twisted and thick-walled, and similar changes occur elsewhere in the body. When the level of oestrogen drops suddenly, bleeding occurs from the womb (menstruation) and thus also precipitates a migraine attack. *Menstrual migraine* is therefore defined as an attack occurring on the day of onset of the menstrual period plus or minus one or two days. If the woman's menstrual periods are regular, oestrogen supplements are given to prevent migraine attacks at this time by decreasing the profound drop in oestrogen levels in the blood.

Oestrogen patches in varying doses (25µg, 50µg and 100µg) can be applied anywhere on the skin three days before the anticipated onset of menstruation. The idea is that the oestrogen levels are prevented from falling rapidly but are not kept so high that they prevent the menstrual period. The danger is that too much oestrogen is used, which prevents further periods. For this reason, the smaller dose patch is prescribed but, if the period does not occur at its usual time and a headache develops, a second skin patch can be applied. This technique – which is meant not to raise the hormonal level but to slow its rapid decrease – can be extremely successful.

Some women have headaches a week before their period; others have them during the last days of their period and yet others get them at the time of ovulation (i.e. midway between the menstrual periods) but these will not respond to the patch technique. Before the menstrual period, women often complain of increased weight due to water retention. This, too, has been associated with migraine attacks, and the disappearance of the attack is often marked by an unusually greater need to pass urine.

Before puberty, the incidence of migraine is equal in girls and boys. After puberty, however, it becomes three times more common in women. This is clearly related to hormonal changes. In adult life, there is a tendency for headaches to get better with increasing age, but this is not consistent and some women may get a worsening of their headaches around the time of the menopause. About 80 per cent of women who suffer from headaches lose them during pregnancy, particularly those who have had menstrual migraine – presumably because the level of oestrogen in the blood remains constant during pregnancy. In others, however, headaches may become worse in early pregnancy.

The 'pill'

Oestrogen given in the first half of the menstrual cycle prevents ovulation and is one basis for the use of oral contraceptives. Headaches may develop soon after starting the first course of the contraceptive pill. They used to be very severe and were sometimes accompanied by signs of malfunction of the nervous system but, with the 'low dose' pill, these are now rare.

Some women taking the pill become severely depressed; this is of interest in the light of the relation between migraine and depression. There is some evidence now that young women who have migraine with aura and take the pill are more likely to have a stroke at a young age, but the overall risk remains small.

Other possible triggers

A well-known precipitant of migraine is air travel. In long-haul journeys this may be due to jet-lag with change in the customary biological rhythms of sleep and wakefulness. Another factor is that, although cabins are pressurised, the ambient pressure is still less than atmospheric; this may well have an effect on the blood vessels in the brain, with dilatation of the small arteries (capillaries).

Many people with migraine are certain that changes in the weather and some winds can trigger attacks. These, too, may be related to changes in barometric pressure but scientific studies have never fully confirmed this explanation.

7
The investigation of headaches

Although nearly everyone has a headache at some time, it is only when the headaches become severe or frequent and interfere with daily living that a doctor's advice is sought. Migraine affects more than one person in five, but only a small percentage of them visit their doctor.

People with headaches are not only concerned with seeking relief but are also often worried whether their headaches mean something more serious, such as a brain tumour. So how do family doctors decide whether a headache is due to migraine or to another cause, and when will they refer a patient to a specialist?

History

The most important aspect of a consultation with the doctor is the taking of a history. With headaches as the chief complaint, the doctor asks about:

- the type of headache,
- how often it happens,
- how long it lasts,
- the site(s) of the pain,
- what brings it on,
- what makes it worse,
- what makes it better,
- any accompanying symptoms such as nausea or visual disturbance,
- previous illnesses,
- the family history.

In most cases a definite diagnosis can be made at this stage, and the physical examination and special investigations will confirm it.

Physical examination

The physical examination can include a general examination of all the body's systems – the pulse is taken, the heart listened to, the blood pressure measured and the abdomen felt.

In a full neurological examination, the cranial nerves are tested one by one. The ability to smell may need to be checked. It is important to test vision, especially visual acuity (using a chart with rows of letters that get ever smaller) and visual fields – the clarity of vision. The ophthalmoscope is an instrument designed to enable the doctor to look at the back of the eye, where the optic nerve, blood vessels and retina can be seen. This is particularly important in people with suspected increased pressure on the brain. Movements of the eyes, the facial and jaw muscles, the soft palate and the shoulders are tested, as are hearing and sensation on the face.

The power of the muscles and sensation in the rest of the body are then tested, as are 'fine' movements and co-ordination – touching each finger with the thumb in sequence. The tendon reflexes at the ankles, knees, elbows and wrists are tested to check that they are equal on both sides. The soles are scratched to ascertain the movement of the big toes, a down-going toe being the normal response. At some stage the doctor will listen over the neck, head and eyes for any murmurs – noises caused by turbulence in blood flow produced by narrowing or malformation of the blood vessels. The head and neck are felt to determine if there is any local tenderness. Difficulties with jaw opening may be a cause of facial pain.

In most cases of headache the examination is negative, suggesting that the cause is probably not serious. Occasionally, though, small changes apparent on the examination may alert the doctor to the possibility of a more serious problem and it is then that the person may be referred to a specialist for investigations.

Special investigations

When nothing definite is found by the examining doctor, requests may be made for every possible test in the hope that something positive will be revealed. This is not only wasteful but also the results, instead of being reassuring, can be misleading. Statistically, the more tests that are done, the greater the number of 'abnormal' results. This produces a vicious circle where a healthy person is investigated extensively at great expense to explain, for example, a chemical abnormality in the blood tests – which could well have been coincidental or irrelevant.

With careful consideration, these disadvantages are avoided. The purpose of special investigations is to provide information beyond that obtained from the history and clinical examination, so it is important to define what questions the doctor hopes to answer. The tests most useful in the diagnosis of a headache can be divided, for convenience, into those of the blood and others.

Blood tests

When a sample of blood is analysed, information is obtained about the state of the blood cells and the fluid (serum) in which they float.

The main cell in the blood is the *red blood corpuscle*, which contains the chemical (haemoglobin) that carries oxygen. The level of haemoglobin can easily be measured. Anaemia occurs when the level of haemoglobin drops but, in some circumstances, there can be too much haemoglobin – the blood becomes thicker and passes through the small vessels less readily, and this may cause vascular problems.

Another important test is the rate at which red blood cells settle when put in a vertical glass tube. This is called the erythrocyte sedimentation rate (ESR). In someone with headache due to an inflammatory disorder such as sinusitis or temporal arteritis (see Chapter 2), the rate of sedimentation will be rapid and produce a high ESR.

Another important type of cell is the *white blood corpuscle*, which helps ward off infection. These cells can be counted easily: a low count means that either there is an abnormality in their production or they are being destroyed too rapidly. A high count occurs during many types of infection; there are several varieties of white blood corpuscle, and the group that is increased indicates the type of infection. This estimate may be of value in, for example, distinguishing a migraine attack, where the white cell count will be normal, from sinusitis, where the count may be higher.

Other special investigations

X-rays

An X-ray of the skull gives only limited information; for example, it will show fractures, sinusitis or inflammation of the bone. A tumour within the skull may be revealed by thinning or thickening of the bone overlying it. Shadows of calcium can be seen in various areas in the skull cavity. They can occur in 'hardening' of the arteries to the brain and, much more rarely, in relatively benign tumours that have been present for a long time. A common place to find calcium shadows is the pineal gland; this is normal but, because the gland is central, a displacement indicates that there is a growth pushing it to one side. These alarming features are virtually never found in someone with migraine. In fact, the skull X-ray of 100 people without headaches would show abnormalities about as often as those of 100 people with migraine. For this reason, a plain X-ray of the skull is rarely done in straightforward migraine. For the same reason, an X-ray of the chest is seldom done unless certain causes of headache are suspected – for example, that a tumour of the lung has spread to the head.

Because headache is sometimes caused by neck trouble, an X-ray of the neck (cervical spine) is sometimes indicated. Although migraine is not usually caused by problems in the neck, wear and tear of the neck vertebrae can cause pain; this in turn results in spasm of the neck muscles, which pull on the scalp and give rise to tension (muscle-contraction) headache. Treatment for this arthritic pain can often relieve these headaches. Pressure on the roots of the cervical nerves also causes pain, particularly over the back of the head.

Electroencephalography (EEG)
Brain cells produce minute fluctuations in electrical current, which can be recorded by placing small metal discs, attached to suitable amplifiers, on various parts of the head. The numerous electrical impulses associated with the living brain tend to produce a particular repetitive pattern. With a person's eyes closed, *alpha rhythm*, consisting of waves lasting one-tenth of a second, occurs; when the eyes are opened the brain is alerted and this rhythm disappears. Faster (*beta*) rhythms may be seen in a person who is using tranquillisers; slower (*theta*) rhythms indicate a malfunction of the brain and even slower (*delta*) rhythms a brain tumour.

Slower rhythms may also be seen in some people with migraine, but many have a normal EEG. EEG findings are never conclusive, because many different abnormalities can give identical EEG changes. A small percentage of 'normal' people without symptoms have EEG changes but they occur more commonly in those with migraine. EEGs are also done in people with migraine if there is any possibility of seizures or blackouts. During one stage of the EEG examination, the person may be asked to 'over-breathe' – to breathe rapidly and deeply. This causes carbon dioxide to be 'blown off', producing a change in the acidity of the blood. Over-breathing can bring out latent abnormalities but, although people with migraine have slightly different responses, these do not necessarily have medical significance.

Another EEG technique to reveal latent abnormalities is the response to a stroboscope, a machine that produces flashing lights (flicker) at different frequencies. In the vast majority of migraine subjects, the responses in the EEG are made to a much greater range of flash frequencies than in people without migraine; however, as a similar phenomenon was observed in those with anxiety and tension who do not suffer from migraine, this too may not be significant.

The EEG can indicate a structural abnormality of the brain but it is not always possible to distinguish one cause from another. Indeed, some deep-seated problems may cause no EEG abnormality or only minimal generalised changes, which can be found in 'normal' people. The EEG supplies a useful piece of the jigsaw puzzle but rarely gives the whole answer on its own.

Rather like the skull X ray, the EEG will reveal something unsuspected only in some instances, when more extensive investigations are indicated.

Evoked potential responses

The EEG machine can also be used to measure the *visual evoked response*. This is a newer technique that is also based on recording electrical activity from the brain. When an object is seen or a sound is heard, an electrical discharge passes along the optic or the auditory pathway, causing a specific but tiny response in the brain – an *evoked response* When the same impulse is presented repeatedly the responses can be added up by an EEG machine to give a much bigger response, shown on a screen in the form of a 'wave' (a wave-form). Using this technique, the time taken for the impulse to travel along the optic or auditory pathway can be measured by taking the time from seeing or hearing the object (the stimulus) to the peak of the wave. Conditions such as inflammation or pressure on the optic or auditory nerve will slow the response, whilst damage to the brain can alter the shape of the wave-form.

Evoked potentials are not generally used in assessing migraine patients. However, early studies performed in the 1970s and 1980s and more recently suggest that people with migraine respond with a larger electrical response. This indicates that the brain of people with migraine reacts to stimuli more strongly than does the brain of people without migraine. Using large numbers of sensing points over the head when performing evoked potential tests produces a 'map' of the brain's electrical activity. This is not useful in routine investigations but it had research potential until overtaken by magnetic resonance imaging (MRI), which is discussed later in this chapter.

CT scanning

Computed tomographic (CT) scanning is quick and easy, and initially revolutionised the diagnosis of neurological disorders. CT scanning examines 'slices' of brain by moving the X-ray machine in such a way that the 'slice' is motionless relative to the areas in front of, and behind, it. The moving areas become blurred while the 'slice' – the area to be examined – retains its sharpness and is defined more clearly. The CT technique depends on the fact that different tissues absorb different amounts of radiation, so it is then easy to identify the different structures to see if there is any abnormality. It is extremely unlikely that a CT scan will reveal any abnormalities in people with migraine who have no other suspicious symptoms. Nevertheless, many patients demand a scan in order to reassure themselves that there is 'nothing bad in there' such as a tumour, an aneurysm or some other abnormality of the blood vessels that could burst and kill them. The preferred imaging technique for these is an MRI scan, discussed below.

MRI scanning

Magnetic resonance imaging (MRI) was introduced in the early 1980s. This technique uses the principle that water, present in all cells, will be affected by a magnetic field. The molecules of water orientate themselves along the line of the magnetic field. If the molecules of water in the magnetic field are disturbed, they will try to get back to their original positions within the field and thus give off energy. The amount of energy and the cells' ability to move can be picked up by sensors and converted into very accurate images of the brain. The technique has revolutionised imaging in much the same way that CT scanning did in the early 1970s. The advantage is that MRI is extremely flexible in that differences in the way that the stimuli apply to the water molecules will cause different aspects of the image to appear. This means that it will show more clearly vascular changes such as alterations in blood vessels or the brain tissues they supply.

MRI is an extremely valuable and powerful tool in the assessment of brain disease. With various modifications in software it is possible to outline all the arteries in the brain (*magnetic resonance angiography*, MRA) to look for any abnormalities in the arteries and to identify areas of abnormal brain tissue. The results can, however, be misinterpreted. When it was first introduced, some migraine patients were diagnosed as having multiple sclerosis on the basis that they had some abnormal areas in the brain (high intensity spots). These lesions in the white matter of the brain, sometimes called 'unidentified bright objects' (UBOs), are present in most people over the age of 40 and seem to be more common in people with migraine. They are such a common finding that they are not regarded as indicating any sinister disease.

Functional magnetic resonance imaging (FMRI) has revolutionised doctors' ability to see function in the nervous system by looking at the blood flow to certain areas of the brain. This technique has revealed that the brains of people who have migraine respond much more actively than the brains of people who do not. For example, a visual stimulus that activates the back part of the brain (the occipital cortex) causes a much greater area of the whole brain to show an increase in blood flow in migraineurs than in non-migraineurs.

Positron emission tomography (PET) is a research technique using radioactive isotopes. When combined with MRI, it can identify areas in the brain that become active when a migraine attack starts. Several centres in the world have identified the area in the brainstem that becomes active during migraine attacks; there is also an area in the part of the brain called the lateral hypothalamus that becomes active during cluster headache attacks. Research on someone who had both types of headache was investigated in this way: when he had a migraine attack the 'migraine generator' lit up on the monitor and when he had a cluster attack the 'cluster generator' lit up. This confirms the view that different types of headache have their sources in different parts of the brain.

Arteriography
Another technique, which relies on the introduction into the blood vessels of substances that can be detected on X-ray (arteriography), may have to be done in order to define the vascular structures more clearly on X-ray films. This has been largely superseded by MRA, as even the vessels at the base of the brain can be visualised and so an injection is not needed.

Ruling out cardiovascular abnormalities

Investigations are important to rule out other abnormalities – for example, an *aneurysm* (a balloon-like distension) found at the junction of two vessels making up the circle of Willis (see Figure 5.4). This can cause headache as well as pressure on sensitive structures in the brain, leading to paralysis of one of the cranial nerves. Small leaks from such an aneurysm, or tiny expansions of it, can cause headaches resembling migraine. If the aneurysm bursts, the resulting bleeding (haemorrhage) can be catastrophic.

Another possible abnormality that can be detected is an *arteriovenous malformation* – a collection of blood vessels rather like the strawberry birthmark seen on the skin. Present from birth, they vary in size and their presence will be suspected if the doctor hears a murmur – the noise of turbulent blood flow. The malformations cause a number of symptoms, including epilepsy or haemorrhage. They may occasionally cause weakness of one side of the body, and can also be associated with a migraine-like syndrome, as in the following case.

Maurice Norton, a 24-year-old man, went to a headache clinic complaining of headache over the right side of his head, with symptoms of classic migraine. Careful examination revealed no abnormality, and the skull X-rays, EEG and brain scan were all normal. The condition was treated as migraine and Maurice responded well. Within a few weeks he collapsed at work, having had a subarachnoid haemorrhage (stroke). Arteriography revealed a small arteriovenous malformation in the front part of the brain. He was operated on, the malformation successfully removed and he had no further headaches.

8
Treatment without drugs

There is no active drug, not even aspirin, that does not have side-effects. It has been estimated that nearly one-third of all illnesses are 'iatrogenic' – they are the unwanted effects of drugs. For this reason, many people would prefer to do without drugs if possible.

People with chronic headaches need a sympathetic doctor who will listen and relate to them. Often, they have seen many doctors who have told them that they should be thankful that they do not have a brain tumour or that they should 'learn to live with it' – the implication being that their benign problems do not warrant more than a few minutes of the doctor's time. On the contrary, not only should they be reassured that they do not have a serious underlying disease but also the cause of their symptoms should be explained. They need information to pass on to their family and teachers or employers, who may not appreciate that the headaches can be disabling and not the more common variety that responds to simple aspirin.

There are two main approaches to the management of migraine: first, prevention and, second, treatment of the symptoms as soon as they occur. Most people with migraine do not go to their GP about it, and many do so only if their symptoms suddenly become more frequent or more severe. This increase in frequency may be due either to an alteration in life circumstances (e.g. increasing stress) or to increased exposure to more specific triggers. There may be a combination of the two; for example, when someone whose headaches are made worse by tobacco smokes more under stress, the combination of these two factors – smoking and stress – is likely to aggravate migraine more than either one singly.

Migraine attacks often cease during pregnancy, which is fortunate as most drugs should be avoided at this time. In contrast, the condition may be worsened by the contraceptive pill, sometimes taking up to a year after its withdrawal to improve.

Preventing migraine attacks

Because primary headaches cannot always be 'cured' in the sense of eliminating them permanently, a reasonable goal is to abort individual headaches and to decrease headache frequency and severity to a degree that does not interfere with normal life. This may be accomplished with medication, with non-drug methods, or both. What is successful for one person may not be for another, so patience is required while the different possibilities are tried. In the search for the most effective treatment, the doctor must be guided by the individual's reports rather than relying only on a physical examination or results of laboratory tests. A patient's confidence in the doctor plays an important part in controlling headaches.

Once the diagnosis of migraine is established, the next step is reassurance – as early as possible – that there is no evidence of any progressive or life-threatening disease. Many people will respond to this alone. The next step is to ascertain if there are any trigger factors. Missing a meal may be a precipitating factor, improvement often following a more regular schedule of eating. Weekend migraine may be due to sleeping later in the morning, so the cure may be achieved by maintaining the same wake-up timetable seven days a week.

Non-drug treatments include counselling, behavioural management, relaxation therapy, biofeedback of various types, hypnotherapy, TENS (transcutaneous electrical nerve stimulation), acupuncture, chiropractic and physiotherapy to the neck. None has been shown by clinical trials to produce any lasting benefit. However, stress is the most common precipitating factor, so, when self-help networks are not taken up and non-drug advice is not effective, there is a place for the temporary use of tranquillisers (see Chapter 9).

Many people report that their attacks are caused by certain foods, particularly cheese, chocolate, oranges and, sometimes, pork. At present there is no scientific evidence for these, although it can be proven scientifically by testing, as has been done with red wine. Others might not have noticed such an association with their headaches, possibly because their attacks have been triggered by other factors arising at the same time. Nevertheless, avoiding particular foods can help greatly, even though there may be no scientific evidence to prove this.

Richard Stephens, a 32-year-old man who was prone to occasional attacks of migraine, suddenly developed terrible headaches that occurred every day. The headaches had all the characteristics of migraine, with nausea and sensitivity to light and sound. When he went on holiday the headache disappeared within two days and he was headache-free during his holiday. Further inquiry revealed that his job, which had recently changed, was to mix sausage meats this involved putting buckets of sodium nitrate into minced meat and mixing them together. As a result, he inhaled a huge amount of nitrate, which was enough to trigger the daily headaches.

When someone starts having daily headaches, it is important to look into any changes in their lifestyle, including changes in their work or housing.

The placebo response

The Latin word *placebo* means 'I will please'. The term 'placebo response' is used to describe a person getting better on treatment that, theoretically, should have no effect at all. This can happen, surprisingly, even with serious illnesses. The symptoms and signs of illness disappear because the person believes that the treatment is helping, demonstrating the close relationship between mind and body. Some types of faith-healing work in this way, fortifying the individual, boosting confidence that something is being done and increasing the body's recuperative powers. There is no doubt that our psychological status affects many of the body's mechanisms.

The placebo response is also influenced to a great extent by the attitude and personality of the attending therapist, and this is illustrated by the following case:

Olivia Pearson, a 30-year-old housewife, had headaches that
were getting worse and happening more often. Her 12-year-
old daughter was having eating problems and Olivia was
becoming increasingly frustrated and angry, and at times she
hit the child. During her first clinic visit, Olivia confided her
problems to a friendly and sympathetic doctor and, by the
end of the interview, was much relieved. A remission from
headaches of several weeks followed. At her next visit, the
doctor who saw her adopted a stern and critical attitude; ten
minutes later, she began to have a severe migraine, which got
better when she was given medication.

Avoidance of stress

Stress is the most common provocative factor, and a logical form
of treatment is to lessen this if at all possible. Frustrating
situations are encountered in nearly all walks of life, as the
following report from someone with migraine demonstrates.

As far as migraine is concerned, the year beginning 1 July
was noteworthy because the attacks were infrequent and
mild. During this period there was enough work to fill the
day comfortably, making it possible for me to maintain
certain personal ideals of perfection. From November the
greatest amount of concentration was given to frequent
short periods of rather monotonous, but not unpleasant,
laboratory work. On 4 February it was suggested that I
attempt to complete my research sufficiently to present an
abstract of the work to a scientific society within 16 days, for
consideration as a presentation at a later date. Accepting this
suggestion, I increased my concentration on this problem by
working in the evenings. It soon became evident that the
amount of work I accomplished was falling far short of any
schedule that would produce enough data by the deadline;
furthermore, the work was, for the first time, becoming
distasteful. The night after my second evening in the
laboratory I was awakened by an ache over my right eye
and I felt sick. After a period of semi-wakefulness, I fell

asleep again and the next day the only trace of a headache was pain on the right side of my head when I coughed. After the third evening of laboratory work I was awakened at 4 a.m. by an ache over my left eye, again feeling sick. Unlike the symptoms of the previous night, they rapidly increased in severity until it became necessary to lie in a hot bath to get some relief. When I returned to bed, the pain and nausea resumed their former severity but 20mg of codeine finally gave me some relief and allowed me a few hours of sleep. Throughout the next day I felt sick and had a constant severe headache that went down into the back of my neck; it was made worse by walking, talking or reaching. The following morning the symptoms had vanished.

This story will strike a chord with almost everyone who has migraine. Although it is possible to explain this sort of tension on chemical changes in the brain, too few studies have been done in situations of chronic stress to pinpoint the problem. Nevertheless, the existence of two different personality types (discussed under 'Stress' in Chapter 6) is pertinent. Type B people who thrive on challenges get a 'charge' or 'kick' by being active and doing things, and may in fact be depressed and lethargic when under-stimulated; with this personality, absence of stress may spark off headaches. The person reported above, however, is an example of a type A personality, who reacted badly to stress.

Although a certain amount of stress is a normal part of human existence, excessive amounts can undoubtedly affect us badly. The first step in lessening stress, which often helps greatly, is to remove any worries about the nature of the headaches by being reassured that there is nothing more seriously wrong. Only very rarely do worries about the nature of the illness need referral to a psychiatrist.

Relaxation

Although lifestyle cannot always be changed, the worsening of any stress-related disorder indicates the need for it to be re-examined. Obvious examples include the person who never takes time off to relax; here the important point is that one headache a month equals one day lost from work each month, so it is a good investment to take time off. Some type A people may not find it helpful to have periods of relaxation (e.g. just staring at the ceiling); the answer might then be physical exercise, starting gently if they are unaccustomed to it.

It is impractical to suggest that someone resign from a demanding job, but it should be possible to find ways to cope with the pressures involved in the work. By preventing the physiological (e.g. hormonal) changes caused by stress, the cycle of chemical changes involved in migraine can be arrested. A useful way to achieve this is relaxation therapy, in which many of the changes induced in the body are the reverse of those seen in the tension headache/migraine syndrome: muscle tone tension in the muscle is decreased, and breathing and the heart rate are slowed. There are numerous types of relaxation therapy: the Japanese communal bath (which is not used for cleansing purposes), the American 'whirlpool' (Jacuzzi) and massage are all attempts in this direction. (A sauna can be helpful but many people find that using it can bring on an attack.) There is considerable evidence that learning to relax helps a tense person reduce the incidence of headaches but it is difficult to separate this improvement from the placebo response, so the claims to success of relaxation therapy are difficult to interpret.

Sometimes the people who most need relaxation find it hardest to achieve. A good way to recognise how tense we are is to consider our posture: a typical example is sitting on the edge of the chair, leaning forward with shoulders hunched and fists clenched. If we hold this posture for a few minutes, we begin to feel discomfort. Where posture is a problem, some people respond to the Alexander technique. Breathing deeply and smoothly helps us to relax but interrupted irregular breathing and sometimes unconsciously holding our breath can indicate that we may be resistant to the idea of relaxation therapy.

Relaxation therapy aims to provide a variety of positive steps to ensure that the last remains of tension have been removed. Relaxation is much easier in a warm, quiet room. Many hospitals and therapists have their own techniques for relaxation, and the summary of such a method given in the Appendix is typical of those currently available.

Meditation

The many different forms of meditation can be grouped into two general categories: those concerned with 'emptying the mind' and those in which internal thoughts are built up and maintained by an effort of concentration.

Transcendental meditation became very fashionable in the West during the 1960s and much is claimed for it by people who have headaches. It is not surprising that relaxing or withdrawing from everyday activities is associated with relief of tension, with consequent reduction in the frequency of headaches. It is less likely to be effective once a headache has started, presumably because the metabolic changes that occur during the headache make it difficult to maintain the appropriate state of mind.

Yoga

Yoga is an ancient Indian technique of achieving total bodily and mental control in an attempt to reach new heights of awareness and in promoting relaxation.

'Yoga of the body' is concerned with making the body a fit vehicle for the mind as it meditates. The first precepts of control are based on the types of food ingested, and is similar to much of the dietary advice often given for migraine – no citrus fruits, little cheese, no alcohol or wine, no garlic or onions and, in addition, no smoking. (Garlic and onions are excluded because they may cause gastric upset.) Meals are taken three times a day, the stomach being 'half filled with food, a quarter filled with water and one quarter left empty' to prevent any feeling of fullness. Food has to be chewed thoroughly and eaten slowly (in contrast to the gulping of quick snack lunches). Constipation is prevented by adding bran to the diet. Much of this advice is common sense and it is understandable that, with this regimen, the body may function better.

Yoga exercises are divided into those in which breathing is the main concern and those that exercise the rest of the body. The breathing exercises are designed to establish conscious control over respiration as well as using the abdominal muscles to ensure that the lungs inflate fully.

The bodily exercises are performed very slowly and involve either stretching movements or maintaining particular positions for periods of time, with relaxation between each posture. Physiologically, maintaining a certain posture uses the stretch reflex of muscles. The whole system can be likened to a cat stretching and rolling, with slow and graceful movements. It is essential that these exercises become comfortable, which needs patience, but, after three months' practice, many people find that they feel better, fitter and much less likely to develop headaches.

There are many techniques for teaching yoga. The meditation aspect of yoga is the most important, so the techniques controlling thought, or holding thoughts in the mind and so building on them, are likely to be of most benefit in developing control.

Psychiatric treatment

Many people with migraine have some degree of depression, but this may be the *result* of their headaches rather than the cause. The opinion of a psychiatrist may prove of value, because their training will help them to assess which person will respond best to which particular therapy. Some experts favour a more complex interpretation of headaches based on psychoanalytic theory but this approach has rarely proved helpful.

The concept of 'co-morbidity' is based on the fact that other conditions seem to be present in the same person more often than by chance. This does not mean that there is a common mechanism or that one condition causes another, although this may be the case. Psychological conditions that may be present in someone with migraine include depression, anxiety or panic attacks.

Biofeedback

Biofeedback is the term used for the method by which we can consciously control automatic functions. This is achieved by the therapist 'feeding back' to the individual information about the automatic function so that its control can be modified. This is usually done by means of either a number on a dial or a tone on a monitor. The person is instructed to achieve a particular number or tone by altering some internal process(es). What this alteration entails is difficult to say, as some people find it almost impossible to specify. They may use a variety of techniques such as imagining themselves on a warm beach or in some other pleasant situation. An example of biofeedback is learning how to ski. It is impossible for the student to say how they stop themselves from falling over but, nevertheless, this eventually occurs and, having happened, is reinforced so that the action becomes natural.

Possibly the most common use of biofeedback is in the control of blood pressure, where people are asked to concentrate in various ways and the results of their efforts are relayed to them; most can learn a technique that will reduce their blood pressure. People with epilepsy often say 'I almost had an attack but I felt it coming and fought it off' – which can be verified using EEG monitoring. They can be taught to suppress epileptic activity when the EEG information is fed back to them, but how this suppression happens is not known.

There have been many attempts to treat migraine in the same way. Three types of information can be relayed to the person with migraine, the first of which is the degree of distension of the temporal artery. This can easily be measured: during an attack of migraine, the temporal artery becomes dilated and the individual can learn to reduce the diameter of the artery, and thus abort attacks.

Muscle contraction can also be brought under feedback control. When a migraine attack associated with neck muscle tension develops, contraction of the neck can be recorded using a machine – the electromyograph (EMG). Therapy consists of feeding back to the person information on the amount of muscle activity in the neck, so encouraging him or her to relax. Results have been fairly encouraging but there is a great placebo effect because there is not a close connection between the feeling of muscle tension and EMG activity; the relief of tension can work by affecting the stress provoking the migraine attack. Other forms of relaxation not using biofeedback can also relieve the tension in the muscles of the neck.

The third use of biofeedback concerns the increase in temperature over the head during a migraine attack with its increase in blood flow; this is most marked during an attack of cluster headache. The response of the blood vessels in the limbs to increased blood flow is abnormal in people with migraine, and increasing the flow of blood through the skin of the hand is associated with a decreased flow of blood to the skin of the forehead. People can alter the blood flow through their hands by concentrating using temperature biofeedback; the dominant hand, which is usually the right hand, shows the best response. Using biofeedback, people can be trained to warm their hands when an attack is coming on. This technique is not effective in everyone, though, because the responses of the blood vessels vary. (Similar responses to the same stimuli occur in anger: some people go white due to constriction of their blood vessels whilst others go red due to dilation of their blood vessels.)

Hand-warming is worth trying, as the biofeedback apparatus needed is fairly simple. It consists of a thermometer attached to the hand and a means of relaying the information to the individual. These devices are becoming commercially available and are not too expensive. The person sits in a relaxed position and tries various thoughts in order to obtain vessel constriction until a satisfactory lessening in blood flow is achieved, as indicated by a small decrease in temperature. It is the skin temperature that is important, so there is no point in clenching the hand. With practice, when the technique has been mastered, changes in temperature of one to two degrees Celsius can be achieved.

Reports from people with headaches who have tried biofeedback successfully bear out the usefulness of the method. For example, one person, who suffered from severe cluster headaches, said 'I know it sounds funny, but I think that if I concentrate I can make my hand feel warmer and then the pain in my head seems to get better.'

Nerve blocks

In recent years many pain clinics have opened where the use of nerve 'blocks' is claimed to have reduced the frequency and severity of headaches, including migraine. The nerve most often blocked is the greater occipital nerve, which comes from the first, second and third nerve roots in the neck (cervical nerve roots C1, C2, C3) and travels to one side of the back of the head. This nerve can be swollen and very tender to touch. The rationale for this block is that reducing the inputs from these nerves into the trigeminal nucleus may reduce the frequency of headaches. The injection to produce the block usually consists of a combination of local anaesthetic and steroid but may be painful. Another substance that may be used is botulinum toxin (Botox), discussed in Chapter 9. If the nerve block procedure is successful, the effect lasts for days, weeks or even months.

There have been few scientific studies that convincingly confirm the effectiveness of nerve blocks but many people given this treatment find them helpful. The problem with evaluating this technique is that those who try it have already tried simpler therapies that failed; this means that they can be the most resistant patients to treat and not respond easily to therapy.

Exercise

Exercise can bring on headaches in some people, but the reverse is also true in that physical training can be of benefit in preventing headaches, by 'toning up' the body and, possibly, the blood vessels. The effect of training on performance is well recognised: the heart and lungs work more efficiently so we do not get out of breath so easily, the blood flow to muscles increases, and the muscles themselves become larger so that we do not get tired as readily. In the trained person, the heart beats more slowly at rest; during exercise, it does not beat as fast as before training nor does the blood pressure rise as high. A greater efficiency is achieved due to increased parasympathetic activity (see Chapter 6): the amount of noradrenaline and adrenaline released for a given amount of exertion decreases; in addition, supplies of energy become more readily available, which also helps to prevent fatigue.

When untrained people first start exercising, the level of glucose in their blood drops, releasing hormones that break down stored supplies of sugar to raise the blood level. In trained people, however, the blood sugar level rises immediately they start exercising. This is because training makes the body more efficient, so it is more able to resist the effects of stress. The result is that people who exercise are able to do more during the day without getting tired.

Studies of the effects of exercise training on the frequency of headaches in people with migraine have had encouraging results. Jogging is the best sort of exercise for this purpose because it moves the greatest bulk of muscle and speeds up the heart rate. You should measure the distance and speed each time, the minimum number of runs being three times a week. It is important to jog fast enough to raise your pulse rate above 150 per minute and for long enough to make you slightly tired.

Acupuncture

The ancient Chinese technique of acupuncture has become popular in the West. Great claims have been made for the technique, particularly in the field of pain relief – for example, in people undergoing major surgery with acupuncture anaesthesia.

The old Chinese teachings state that the body consists of a balance of positive and negative forces – the *yin* and the *yang* – that flow through various channels in the body, along which there are special points where the flow can be influenced. Particular points are thought to relate to specific organs. The acupuncturist feels many acupuncture 'pulses' and, through abnormalities in these, arrives at a diagnosis. Inserting sharp needles into the appropriate combination of points is claimed to stop pain, as well as producing healing, in a particular organ.

There is no doubt that this technique can work as far as pain relief is concerned, but the evidence that it influences healing of disease is dubious. The theory has no scientific basis – no one has demonstrated the system of channels and points that are meant to cover the body, although there are areas of the skin (corresponding to acupuncture points) where their ability to conduct electricity can be altered. However, it is now known that, after acupuncture, pain-killing substances – endorphins – are released in the brain, and it is this mechanism that provides the scientific basis for acupuncture.

We are left with the question as to how pain is relieved. Legend has it that acupuncture was evolved following the observation by a soldier that the pain of his wound was relieved when he had been pierced by an arrow elsewhere in his body. The explanation might be that, in the heat of battle, adrenaline, noradrenaline and cortisol are released into the blood stream; there is also increased release of chemicals in the brain called opioids, particularly those involved in the appreciation of pain. This could explain how the body feels less pain when geared for a fight. The arrow wound could act not only by its effect of further increasing the release of the pain-reducing substances but also by affecting the 'gating' mechanism for pain. This theory – that there is a 'gating' mechanism in the spinal cord which can either be open, allowing painful impulses to travel up the spinal cord, or shut, to block them – explains how transmission of other sensations can block pain impulses, preventing them from reaching our consciousness. In effect, the pain gate can be shut by other sensations.

Acupuncture may work through similar mechanisms, although exactly how it does this is not known. Sometimes it needs to be fairly painful to be effective and, in some acupuncture centres, a modified form of acupuncture is used passing a small electric current down the needles.

Counter-irritation

Similar in effect to acupuncture are various techniques that employ 'counter-irritation' of the painful area. Some techniques use vibration, in which the person stimulates the painful area for a few minutes each day; others use an electrical shock such as TENS (transcutaneous electrical nerve stimulation) to the affected area. The efficacy of these techniques has yet to be assessed, particularly as they carry a potent placebo effect.

Manipulation

Manipulation of the spine, which can help backache, has been tried with people who have migraine. The theory is that the pain arising at the back of the neck is brought about by malfunction or misalignment of that part of the spine (the cervical spine). No 'controlled' trials have been done, so the theoretical basis for this treatment is not scientifically proven.

Chiropractic

In several developed countries the first thought of those with a headache is to go to a chiropractor. A chiropractor manipulates the spine, especially the neck, with good results for some; there has been no double-blind, placebo-controlled study of chiropractic but it does make anatomical sense. The upper cervical nerves (C1 and C2) have their relay with that part of the spinal cord that carries pain impulses to the brain. The trigeminal nucleus controls the fifth cranial nerve, which is the main sensory nerve of the head. (As mentioned in Chapter 5, this is part of the trigemino-vascular network, which is the 'instrument' by which migraine is generated. Inputs from the cervical spinal cord could activate the trigeminal nucleus – the cervico-trigeminal relay – to produce a headache, possibly including migraine.) It is claimed that some of the beneficial effects are achieved by realigning the bones but this has not been scientifically proven.

Osteopathy

Osteopathy is also based on spinal manipulation. Osteopaths believe that bad posture is the cause of a whole host of disorders – for example, disorders of digestion. Osteopaths are now recognised in the UK by a statutory regulatory body that requires osteopaths to have certain training and standards. In the USA their position is accepted as equivalent to doctors; many medical schools there have recognised departments of osteopathy, and the course of studies is similar in length and content to that required for a medical degree.

Although many of the claims for manipulation are exaggerated, it does have a place in treating certain conditions of the neck that produce headache – by relieving muscle tension. The question of whether there is realignment of bones is more controversial. The practitioner must take care, because the condition can be made worse, in particular because two vertebral arteries run through the spine in the neck to supply the base of the brain; manipulation can lead to the blockage of these vessels, causing a stroke.

Although many people with migraine claim to have obtained relief with osteopathic treatment, there is no clear-cut proof that this method has any greater success than would be expected from the placebo response.

Treatment of allergy

The term 'allergy' is often used to describe an unusual sensitivity but, strictly speaking, it should be used only for an abnormal or inappropriate reaction by the body's immune system to some-thing that would usually be harmless.

Some people get headaches in response to an allergic reaction, possibly due to the release of histamine in the body. Because food allergy seems to play a part in producing some migraine headaches, attempts have been made to desensitise people to the relevant substances. This involves testing for allergy by using small amounts of suspect materials and noting any to which there is a response. The substance is then prepared in minute concentrations and increasing amounts are injected under the skin at frequent intervals in order to increase the body's tolerance to it. This approach works well in hay-fever and some cases of asthma, where there are definite identifiable allergic responses, but the situation in migraine is not as clear-cut. Although some people with migraine have demonstrable food allergy, desensitising them to the offending food does not always achieve any benefit. We need further trials of this form of treatment in a large number of people, comparing the results with those in another group of people who had been 'desensitised' with an ineffective substance. This sort of trial has not yet been undertaken. Nevertheless, if you have a proven allergy to a particular substance, you might derive some benefit from desensitisation; seek advice from a specialist in that area.

Keeping a headache or migraine diary and recording possible triggers is essential to pinpoint possible causes.

Herbal remedies

In Europe, especially Germany, herbal remedies are the favourite treatment for many ills. In some countries they are pre-scribed by doctors in the same way as other medicines. If you are interested in examining the effectiveness of any of the non-drug or alternative treatments, the Bandolier website is extremely valuable. This group from Oxford University post the results of trials of alternative treatments and offer a critical review of the methods used in the trials. This enables us to at least get some concept of what can be tried. However, many so-called natural remedies are not harmless; for instance, some 'bush teas' can cause cirrhosis of the liver. Moreover, it can be difficult to be certain of the quality of the herbs; it can vary according to where the plants were grown and when they were harvested. There have been reports of serious illness and even death resulting from taking herbal remedies – Western as well as Chinese. So anyone giving herbal treatment should be fully trained in this aspect of therapy.

Feverfew

The plant feverfew (Latin name *Chrysanthemum parthenium*) – a hardy perennial, originally from Turkey – has been used for many years in the prevention of migraine attacks. The leaves are harvested when the plant is in flower and contain a variety of chemicals; the ones thought to be active in migraine are known as sesquiterpene lactones, of which parthenolide is one. Many products quote the concentration of parthenolide in the tablet because this particular compound is the most stable. Most of the feverfew in Europe is grown on the Golan Heights and many growers are breeding the plant for higher content of parthenolide. The problem is that we do not know if parthenolide is the active component. Certainly the sesquiterpene lactones have an effect in blocking the re-uptake of serotonin in platelets, and may have an effect like this in the brain.

The other compounds in feverfew are tanetin, which has an anti-lucitrian activity, and the flavonoid compounds. Trials comparing the results of feverfew against a placebo have varied in their results but many people with migraine still use feverfew and swear by its efficacy. Some grow the plant in their gardens and use two fresh leaves twice a day with bread and sugar. If stored, the plants are collected in summer, dried and kept away from damp and sunlight. The leaves are quite bitter and can cause mouth ulcers but standardised tablets are now available in healthfood shops. It is important to use plants of the European variety of feverfew, not the North American variety (known in Mexico as Santamaria) which has no sesquiterpene lactones and is probably ineffective in migraine.

To prevent migraine, either the pure leaf or the leaf extract can be used, given as capsules. The former capsule contains 380mg of pure leaf and is taken three times a day; the latter contains 100mg of leaf extract and is taken only once daily. Both types of capsule should be taken with food.

Feverfew should not be used by anyone taking the contraceptive pill, during pregnancy or breastfeeding. It can cause stomach problems and should not be used for more than four months at a time (to prevent allergic reactions); stopping should be done gradually.

St John's wort and butterbur

St John's wort can be effective in depression but no reliable scientific studies have investigated its value in migraine. As with feverfew, many people find it useful. It can, however, interact with some drugs (e.g. the contraceptive pill), so should not be taken without first discussing the matter with the doctor or pharmacist.

There is also some evidence for the efficacy of butterbur.

Vitamins

Possibly the most interesting non-drug treatment is riboflavin, or vitamin B_2. (Vitamins are essential compounds used in metabolic processes but which are not produced by the body.) The value of B_2 was discovered some years ago by Italian researchers performing magnetic resonance spectroscopy – a technique for looking at the chemical compounds in the body. They found that the chemical changes during muscle usage are reduced in people with migraine. This led to using vitamin B_2, a 'coenzyme', or 'helper' enzyme for the system of energy-producing enzymes. These are present in organelles, called mitochondria, located in muscle cells that produce energy for the body. A preliminary study found that it was effective in reducing the frequency of headaches, and a double-blind, placebo-controlled study (see Chapter 9) confirmed this.

In many headache clinics vitamin B_2 is a standard first-try therapy for people who want a preventive (prophylaxis) without the side-effects associated with drugs. The only side-effect of B_2 is that it turns the urine bright yellow!

When a headache strikes

People with migraine cannot hope to lose all their headaches unless they are extremely lucky – at some stage many treatments fail. It is advisable to take various precautions to avert an attack or to make life tolerable if an attack strikes. Valerie South in her excellent book *Help for Headaches* makes several recommendations:

- Have spare pairs of sunglasses – in the car, at home, in the office – in case it gets very bright; glare is a very frequent cause of headaches.
- If you usually do the family cooking, prepare food in advance and keep it in the freezer to be used when you can't cope.
- Keep bags of peas in the freezer to use as ice-packs.
- If cold doesn't help, warmth can be effective.

Physical methods of treatment during the migraine attack

With infrequent or mild attacks, cutting short the attack is all that is necessary. A variety of treatments are available and, although most are based on the use of drugs (see Chapter 9), some are physical.

A simple way to achieve relief is to press on the temporal artery on each side of the head for several minutes. This reduces the pulsating pain and may cause the arteries to constrict (vaso-constriction). Applying an ice-pack to the head or immersing the head in a cold bath or basin may help, by the same mechanism of vasoconstriction. Ice-packs designed for this purpose are now available from chemist/pharmacist shops; alternatively, a plastic envelope filled with a gel that keeps cold for a long time can be kept in a refrigerator or freezer and used when needed. Because they can warm up relatively quickly, it is worth having more than one of these. Not everyone responds to cold, though, finding warmth more effective.

Other people find that putting their feet into hot water or lying in a hot bath can help, because this also results in vasoconstriction of the scalp. Temperature biofeedback, or hand-warming (as discussed earlier in this chapter), has been tried in this context with some success.

The two time-honoured measures for relief are a darkened room and sleep. They can be as helpful as drugs, which are discussed in Chapter 9.

The methods described in this chapter are extremely important as they are used by almost everybody with migraine at some stage. If a particular method helps, it is certainly worth using it provided that it is not harmful.

9
Treatment with drugs

Clinical trials of new drugs

Before a drug is licensed for use it must undergo rigorous tests, the final one being for people to try it – clinical trials. An important aspect of clinical trials is eliminating the placebo response in which the person expects to get better and does so, despite being given a dummy pill (the placebo). Because we can be influenced by the attitude of the doctor or therapist, it is important that the doctors as well as the patients do not know who is receiving which treatment – the drug being tested or the placebo; this is known as a double-blind trial. Patients are placed randomly either in the group receiving the treatment under trial or in the placebo group. A variety of selection techniques are used to make sure that the mix in both groups is equivalent. This sort of test is called a double-blind, placebo-controlled, randomised trial, and it is the 'gold standard' for testing effectiveness and safety.

The information about who is receiving what is entrusted to a third person who has no influence or contact with the running of the trial. For safety reasons, it is important that somebody knows what is being given so that, if a patient has a problem due either to the treatment or to other factors, the 'blind can be broken' and appropriate action taken.

At the end of the trial the results are analysed by groups. In certain types of trials a safety committee will look at the results without knowing which groups are which. If there is a significant trend that differentiates one group from another, either in terms of effect (control of migraine) or side-effects (untoward symptoms from the drug), the committee has the right to halt the trial and to have the results analysed.

The placebo effect

The placebo effect is described in Chapter 8 but, briefly, it refers to the improvement achieved because the patient receiving the placebo – the dummy pill – expects it to have a beneficial effect, not knowing that there is no 'active' ingredient in it. The following case exemplifies this.

> *Gwithian Rosen, a 44-year-old woman, had frequent migraine attacks. She was given a box of placebo pills with words of kindness, reassurance and indications of great interest. It was also emphasised that she had no serious structural defect or tumour, and she left the clinic feeling relaxed and secure. For six weeks after the interview she was headache free but gradually the condition began to creep back.*

This case history exemplifies a characteristic of migraine. It is quite common for someone with migraine to respond very well initially to any new treatment, but it is nearly as common for the headaches to return later as badly as ever. The explanation is that the initial placebo response wears off and indicates that the treatment has had no specific effect of its own. Another interesting feature is the amazing variety of drugs that seem to be effective in treating migraine. It is for this reason that claims of success for a particular form of treatment have to be analysed carefully. The more attention and interest a person gets, the greater the placebo effect will be. To some extent this may explain the good effect of certain dietary treatment or, indeed, any treatment in which the person obtains a good deal of attention.

A recent example of this was published in the journal *Headache*. During a clinical trial patients who should have received the 'active' medication inadvertently received placebo, because the boxes got mixed up. The investigators documented the effectiveness of this placebo and the effect was at least 40 per cent reduction in severity of attacks, for up to two months. Advocates for particular treatments may publish affidavits from satisfied patients but they are unlikely to publish comments from patients who have *not* responded!

Taking drugs

The difference in drug usage between countries is of interest, and even the way the drug is administered varies widely. In general, the French prefer suppositories, the Italians injections, whilst drops are used in Poland. One possible explanation is that differences in dietary habits may influence the absorption and action of medication.

Most people are reluctant to take drugs. The two main reasons for this are worries about side-effects and worries about becoming dependent on the drugs.

Side-effects

There are very few medicines that are entirely free from unwanted effects. If a drug works, it does so by acting on the body's tissues – so, when too much is taken, it will be harmful. Individuals vary in their reactions, and some are more sensitive than others. Even the most common drugs can produce unpleasant effects – for example, aspirin can result in vomiting of blood in certain individuals if it damages the stomach lining, causing ulcers.

Dependence

Many drugs, particularly those having effects on the brain, such as sedatives and tranquillisers, have the reputation of causing dependence. This means that when the drug is stopped, the individual suffers from unpleasant withdrawal symptoms. The best-known of these are seen in chronic alcoholics and morphine addicts who, when their drug intake is suddenly stopped, develop hallucinations and tremor (trembling or shaking).

In chronic or recurrent disease, of which migraine is one example, it is particularly important to prevent dependence. The withdrawal symptoms experienced after long-term use of sedatives or tranquillisers are comparatively mild but can lead to insomnia, irritability and depression. For these reasons, drugs should be taken only when necessary – when attacks are severe and interfere with daily life. When attacks are frequent, drug therapy may be more effective if preventive (prophylactic) treatment is given rather than waiting for the attacks which, when started, may not be remedied so easily.

Most people with migraine have mild attacks and they usually cope without going to the doctor. It is only when the migraine attacks are severe, and are not controlled by the usual simple measures, that treatment becomes a problem.

Treatment of the attack

The first phase of a migraine attack – the aura – has been considered to be due to constriction of blood vessels to the brain (vasoconstriction of the intracranial circulation). To prevent any possibility of damage to the brain from poor blood flow (cerebral ischaemia), migraine attacks should be prevented before this phase because, once the first symptoms appear, vasoconstriction may have already begun. Although the migraine aura need not be very troublesome in itself, if it is prevented, so is the full-blown attack. Even before the aura, there may be warning signs (prodromal feelings) the day before an impending attack. These are sometimes related to gastric upsets; for example, some people feel hungry, and eating sugar may prevent a worsening of symptoms. The aim is always to stop the headache coming and to prevent nausea and vomiting.

Pain itself has an effect on the blood vessels to the brain – even mild pain causes activity in the area of brain representing the painful area of the body, with a slight increase in blood flow to that region. As pain increases, there is a more general increase in blood flow throughout the whole brain, caused by widening of the blood vessels (vasodilation), which in turn may cause more pain. This cycle can be stopped by using pain-killers to diminish the appreciation of pain; the cycle of pain giving vascular changes giving more pain can also be interrupted by sedation with tranquillisers such as diazepam (Valium). Vasodilation can also be reversed using a short-acting vasoconstricting substance such as one of the triptans (see later).

Not only are nausea and vomiting disturbing in themselves but they also prevent remedies taken by mouth from having an effect. These symptoms are partly due to a chemical messenger (neurotransmitter) acting on the 'vomiting centre' of the brain so that the action of the stomach muscle becomes sluggish (gastric stasis). This means that the contents of the stomach – including tablets – do not readily pass down into the small intestine, where most foods and medicines are absorbed. Unless they are taken early in an attack, before gastric stasis has developed, tablets taken during an attack of migraine do not help because they do not get into the blood stream. Hence the complaint: 'Nothing helps the attacks, I just have to lie quietly in a darkened room and wait for it all to go away.'

During a migraine attack, most people prefer to lie down (although, less commonly, it can make the symptoms worse). The benefit felt is partly because it is difficult to function or concentrate during this time and also because lying down provides some relief from the headache and nausea in most people. Because sound and light are upsetting, a quiet darkened room is preferred. Perhaps the most effective remedy is sleep; on awakening, the symptoms can be much relieved.

Pain-killers (analgesics)

Because one of the best treatments for headache has been a pain-killer, different types of these drugs have been used to stop the pain. The most commonly used pain-killers, such as aspirin or ibuprofen (non-steroidal anti-inflammatory drugs, NSAIDs) or paracetamol, work through their actions on the brain, dulling the perception of pain. Ibuprofen is also available in 'melt' formulation, and is absorbed in the mouth. The stronger NSAIDs that are available only on prescription can be very effective.

If the pain-killer is taken early enough, many people find that this will stop an attack. Because absorption into the blood stream during a migraine attack is variable, it is better to take a soluble or effervescent form of these drugs – particularly if there are stomach problems such as ulcers, which are more likely to be aggravated by non-soluble aspirin tablets. In these instances, antacid preparations may be added to prevent indigestion.

Some people who do not respond well to the triptans or in whom they are contra-indicated may need opiates. Stronger analgesics act directly on the nerve (endorphin) receptors in the brain, making it less responsive to pain. Because most of these drugs are derivatives of opium, they often cause drowsiness or euphoria and sometimes nausea; they include pentazocine, pethidine, codeine, dihydrocodeine, morphine and heroin. The last two should never be used in migraine because of the danger of addiction. Many people find codeine useful, particularly if care is taken to prevent habituation (addiction) to these drugs. The general view is that opiates are best avoided because they are implicated in exacerbations of chronic daily headache.

Anti-emetics

Another useful combination is an analgesic with an anti-emetic – a drug that prevents nausea. Although there are many drugs that act against nausea, only metoclopramide and domperidone also affect the action (motility) of the stomach, making it empty faster so that tablets or medicine will be passed into the small intestine and absorbed more quickly. (This has been shown by measuring the levels of aspirin in the blood stream, which are twice as high when metoclopramide is added during a migraine attack.) To help their absorption the anti-emetic should be taken 15 minutes before other drugs. Although prochlorperazine has a more powerful anti-nausea effect, it does not affect the motility of the stomach. Anti-emetics are more effective when given by injection but this is not always practicable at home or at work. Some people prefer taking these medicines in the form of a syrup. Metoclopramide tablets may not be absorbed and it is not available in suppository form, but domperidone is.

One of the most commonly used remedies for migraine is the combination of an anti-emetic, paracetamol, caffeine and codeine known as Migraleve. Although useful in a mild attack, it is not absorbed rapidly enough to treat severe attacks.

Ergotamine

Some of the most effective remedies in the past have been drugs containing ergotamine, which comes from a mould that grows on rye. The name is derived from the French word *ergot*, meaning a 'spur', because part of the rye fungus resembles a riding spur in shape. Eating bread made from mouldy rye can be poisonous, producing painful blue hands and feet ('St Anthony's fire'). In the Middle Ages, whole villages in Eastern Europe that had been poisoned with the mouldy bread were reported to have been visited by the devil. They were 'cured' by visiting St Anthony's shrine that was in Egypt and therefore well outside the infected area.

Like many other drugs used in the past, the way this compound worked was unknown for many years. Its use in the treatment of headache was first reported in Germany in 1883. In 1889, Dr W Thompson of the USA advised taking fluid extract of ergot by mouth but also suggested that administration into the rectum could be useful:

> As nausea is such a general accompaniment of this affection it is prescribed that if either of the doses be vomited it should be taken in an enema of two ounces of water. This medication rarely fails to arrest the attacks.

After this report, the use of ergot was forgotten, possibly because of the inconsistent effect of the extracts. Then, in 1906, ergotoxine – an extract from ergot – was found, which was later determined to be a mixture of compounds. In 1918 a single substance was isolated – ergotamine – which was originally used to speed up contractions of the uterus during labour (ergot derivatives are still occasionally used in obstetrics). In 1925 ergotamine in its pure form was first used in the treatment of migraine and began to be prescribed widely. But it was not until 1937, when the cause of the migraine headache was ascribed to blood vessels in the head becoming wider (extracranial vasodilation), that it was thought that ergotamine worked by narrowing these blood vessels (vasoconstriction). If the migraine aura was due to vasoconstriction, it was theoretically worrying to give a powerful vasoconstrictor drug; however, there is no lessening of cerebral blood flow.

Ergotamine is usually safe and effective in an acute attack, provided it is given in the correct dosage. Because tablets taken during an attack may not be completely absorbed from the stomach, the timing of the medication is critical.

Other vasoconstricting substances, such as caffeine, have been added to ergotamine, a combination that can make a tablet almost as effective as an injection. Another compound commonly added to ergotamine is a substance against nausea and vomiting (e.g. cyclizine). For some people who have infrequent attacks, the combination is effective and remains their preferred treatment.

Because ergotamine is poorly absorbed when taken in tablet form, it can be given by inhalation or by suppository. When vomiting is a problem, using a suppository can be effective. (An injection is more effective but is no longer available in the UK; outside the UK, the injection is usually given by a doctor but can be self-administered.) When ergotamine is given via an inhaler, a measured dose is administered; this gives rapid absorption and overcomes the twin problems of vomiting and overdosage but the method is not popular, largely because it may give a bad taste.

Because ergotamine is a potentially addictive drug with adverse effects, care is taken to avoid frequent dosing and is no longer given to individuals with frequent attacks. About half the people who take ergotamine have some sort of adverse reaction, such as nausea, shaking, trembling and feeling weak. Signs of ergotamine overdose include chronic background headache with continuous nausea, made worse by increasing the usual dose. These side-effects can be so unpleasant as to make some individuals prefer the migraine symptoms. Because of these problems, ergotamine is no longer the preferred treatment in the UK for a migraine attack.

For people with only occasional attacks of migraine – say, about once every four months – ergotamine is still used. The maximum number of tablets allowed is four tablets in 24 hours or six tablets in a week; this has resulted in the virtual disappearance of hallucinations.

Ergot is related chemically to the powerful hallucinogenic drug lysergic acid diethylamide (LSD), so it is not surprising that other side-effects of ergot occasionally include hallucinations and psychosis.

The chief side-effect now seen from taking ergotamine too often for too long is headache, although this can take more than two weeks to develop. This side-effect has been misinterpreted as being due to further migraine attacks, and so more ergotamine is taken. The headache of ergotamine overdosage is dull and persistent rather than the episodic throbbing character of true migraine, and is not relieved by pain-killers. With ergotamine overdosage, stopping the drug leads initially to a worsening of the headache, but perseverance with not taking the drug will almost always eventually lead to relief from this type of headache. It can take two weeks or more of abstention before the person feels better and the situation is stabilised. It is difficult to break the habit of this particular form of ergotamine addiction or 'habituation', so, to prevent this vicious circle, ergotamine preparations are no longer given if migraine attacks are frequent.

Dihydroergotamine

This is effective during an acute attack but has less vasoconstrictive effect than ergotamine. It became available in 1943 but is no longer used in the UK.

The triptans*

There is now no doubt, since the introduction of sumatriptan in the UK in 1991, that the most effective medication for the treatment of the acute attacks are the triptans. These new drugs for migraine have appeared in a relatively short time. Sumatriptan is by far the best established, and has been effective and safe in large numbers of patients since it was introduced. Which triptan to take will be based on such considerations as the characteristics of each individual's attacks, how well they respond to and tolerate a particular triptan, how well the symptoms other than pain are relieved, the tendency for attacks to recur, how consistently the drug works and which one the individual prefers. Because the clinical trials involved young adults and older, the triptans are not recommended for anyone under the age of 18.

The triptans now available are listed in Table 9.1 and discussed more fully below. Sumatriptan, being the first triptan to be used, is discussed first; the rest are given in alphabetical order.

Sumatriptan
Sumatriptan was the first of this class of compounds called the triptans to be released to treat migraine attacks. It had been the subject of a huge number of studies – indeed, more studies than

*Reproduced, with amendments and additions, from the chapter by Marek Gawel in *Migraine* by Valerie South, by kind permission of the publishers, Key Porter Books Ltd, Toronto.

Table 9.1 Triptans

Generic name	Trade name	Dose
By mouth		
Almotriptan	Almogram	12.5mg
Eletriptan	Relpax	20mg or 40mg
Frovatriptan	Migard	2.5mg
Naratriptan	Naramig	2.5mg
Rizatriptan	Maxalt	5mg or 10mg
Sumatriptan	Imigran	50mg or 100mg
Zolmitriptan	Zomig	2.5mg
Nasal spray		
Sumatriptan	Imigran	10mg or 20mg
Zolmitriptan	Zomig	5mg
Injection		
Sumatriptan	Imigran	6mg
On or under tongue		
Rizatriptan	Maxalt Melt	10mg
Zolmitriptan	Zomig Rapimelt	2.5mg

had ever been done on any compound for migraine prior to this. It was found that sumatriptan stimulated the receptors known as 5-HT$_{1B}$ receptors, which lie on the blood vessels and cause their constriction, and 5-HT$_{1D}$ receptors, which lie on the nerves and cause a release of inflammatory substances. Because 5-HT (5-hydroxytryptamine) is also known as serotonin, many people mistakenly think that these drugs have an effect on the levels of serotonin. The serotonin levels may or may not change but what is actually happening is that receptors 'unlocked' by serotonin are being 'unlocked' by the triptan. With the introduction of sumatriptan, many people found relief from their headaches for the first time.

The first trials of sumatriptan were begun in 1986, the compound being given by injection under the skin (subcutaneously). The clinical trials showed that its use in migraine was extremely effective, and it became available for use in the UK in 1991 (in Canada in 1992, in the USA in 1993). The drug then underwent trials for oral use. It quickly found a place in the treatment of migraine for which it is now the best-selling medication in the world.

Initially, sumatriptan was associated with a number of side-effects – some people developed chest pains and there were even a few reported cases of heart attack following its use. There does not seem to have been much problem in this regard recently, possibly because there is a better understanding of which people should not use the drug. The triptans have some effect on the blood vessels in the heart as well as in the head. Chest tightness and tightness or heaviness in the throat, neck or jaw are common side-effects of most of the triptan group. Triptans may also cause tiredness, sleepiness, nausea, tingling in the hands and feet, and a variety of other problems such as dizziness. But these side-effects do not occur in most people; when they do, they are seldom severe and are very transitory.

After the introduction of oral sumatriptan it became evident that, for most people, a 50mg tablet was as effective as 100mg, and was better tolerated. The official dose is now 50mg, to a maximum of 300mg in 24 hours.

Intranasal sumatriptan is taken in a 20mg dose (maximum 40mg in 24 hours). It is quite effective but some people don't like substances in their nose, and some develop a bad taste as the preparation goes down into their mouth. Ideally, nasal preparations should be absorbed through the mucous membranes inside the nose, at its top, where the membranes are particularly thin. In practice this is difficult to achieve, but they can be useful for people who cannot take tablets by mouth because of nausea and vomiting. Its disadvantage is its greater cost than the tablet, although not of the injection.

Sumatriptan is still the only triptan available for injection. The dose is 6mg and is self-injected under the skin. There is a leaflet explaining simply how to do it and, once used, it is simple to do (world-wide, millions of people with diabetes use self-injection easily every day). Its advantage is that it works within 15 minutes, at whatever stage of an attack it is taken.

Almotriptan
This triptan is taken as a 12.5mg tablet. It can be repeated after two hours if the headache does not go but the maximum dose is two tablets in 24 hours.

Eletriptan

The dose is 40mg, swallowed in water, which can be repeated for a recurrence but not for the same attack. Not more than 80mg should be taken in 24 hours.

Frovatriptan

This is the most recently introduced triptan in the UK. The dose is 2.5mg, and the drug is claimed to have a more prolonged effect.

Naratriptan

Naratriptan (Naramig) has slightly different properties from the other triptans in that it is slightly slower to take effect and seems to last longer so there is less chance of the headache recurring quickly. Although its overall efficacy is not as good as that of the other triptans, many people with migraine prefer it, especially if their headaches start slowly and last a long time. The dose is 2.5mg, which may be repeated after 4 hours (maximum 5mg in 24 hours).

A 1mg dose is being studied as a preventive for menstrual migraine; it is too early to say whether this will be effective, although early studies have been encouraging.

Rizatriptan

This triptan seems to be more effective against nausea than the other triptans. The dose is 10mg; it should not be repeated if the headache doesn't go away but a further 5mg or 10mg can be taken if the headache goes and then returns (maximum of 20mg in 24 hours). It should not be taken until 24 hours after an ergotamine-type drug (and ergotamine should not be taken until six hours after rizatriptan). Rizatriptan is also available in the UK as a 'melt' to be dissolved on the tongue. People taking propranolol should use the 5mg dosage.

Zolmitriptan

Zolmitriptan (Zomig) acts quite rapidly but its side-effects are similar to those of sumatriptan. The dose is 2.5mg, which can be repeated after two hours. It can be increased to 5mg if the lower dose doesn't give relief or for subsequent attacks, to a maximum of 15mg in 24 hours. It is available as a nasal spray, in 5mg doses.

Studies have been done of the nasal spray and of the 'melt' – a rapidly dispersible tablet with an orange taste that is sucked on or under the tongue. It is now available in the UK and Canada.

Note that no triptan is effective in stopping a migraine aura, the mechanism of which is quite different from the other features of a migraine attack.

Regular overuse of triptans, as with other drugs, can lead to problems. The most common is the rebound or medication-induced headache: headaches may start coming back as soon as the medication wears off. It is unwise to regularly use more than about 12 triptan tablets in a month. If headaches occur more often than this, preventive drugs should be considered.

In clinical trials, the severity of headaches has been classified into four categories: severe, moderate, mild or none. To determine whether someone has responded to a drug, the headaches are assessed as to whether they have moved from the 'severe' or 'moderate' categories to the 'mild' or 'none' categories. The usual time-frame for a response is two hours, but in more recent trials earlier responses have been registered as well.

Of course, people would rather not have any headache at all, and the final measure should be 'pain-free'. In practice, however, it is useful to look at reduction of the headaches to mild, because this allows people to continue day-to-day activities without much hindrance. Fixing hopes on a magically symptom-free state would result in disappointing success rates.

People who do not respond well to one of the triptans, or do not tolerate one, should certainly try another, and if necessary a third. Studies have revealed that, even if the response to the first drug is poor, there is a 75 per cent chance of a good response to the second one, and a 15 per cent chance of a good response to the third. Over all, the triptans benefit at least 70–80 per cent of people, and they have had a dramatic impact on the quality of life in numerous people who had previously been disabled by migraine attacks.

Nevertheless, there are some for whom this class of drug does not work or in whom it should not be used; for example, those with a history of heart disease, angina, high blood pressure or other circulatory problems. Some people choose not to take triptans because of adverse effects such as chest or throat tightness and feelings of tiredness, preferring to use more traditional forms of treatment

Not treating the headache

Many people with migraine feel that their attack is 'something from outside', and that calming down the headache merely postpones the development of the full cycle. They feel that preventing vomiting only prolongs the time they feel sick and that it is only after they vomit that they start to feel better; in these circumstances, treatment may just prolong the suffering. The mechanism of such a reaction could be explained by a long-lasting chemical change lurking in the background, which must be allowed to settle naturally It is only by careful study that the truth of this contention will be proven scientifically and the basis of the cyclical nature of migraine understood.

Preventive drugs

There are many types of drugs that can prevent migraine attacks. This indicates not only that migraine is highly complex, with many stages at which prevention is possible, but also that no single drug is necessarily much better than the others. No two people with migraine are the same, and each one needs to be treated as an individual. It may be necessary to try a variety of drugs in order to find which one is most suitable.

Preventive medication is given only for frequent attacks – for example, two or more attacks per month. Because the tablets have to be taken every day, there is no indication for them if the attacks are less frequent, particularly if they are mild or respond well to simple remedies. Only if attacks are interfering with life's ordinary activities should daily preventive tablets be considered to restore a normal life.

Preventive drugs are recommended if attacks are interfering with daily life:

- two or more severe attacks per month, each affecting the person for three or more days,

- frequent, though milder, attacks (e.g. two a week, each lasting up to a day).

They are also used if there are problems with the treatments for the attacks, such as:

- there are contra-indications to their use (e.g. beta-blockers in people with low blood pressure),
- their side-effects are troublesome,
- they don't work,
- too much has been taken.

Other considerations include special circumstances (e.g. hemiplegic migraine) and the individual's preference of wishing to be as free from as many attacks as possible.

Preventive drugs obtained on prescription

These drugs are listed in Table 9.2. They are started at a low dose and increased slowly until there is a good response, unless there are unacceptable side-effects or the full dose is reached. They should be used for at least three months; improvement is noticed in the first month but continues for a further two months, even at the same dosage. Preventive migraine drugs are not meant to be taken for life, just for courses. If the headaches are fully controlled for six months, the improvement will continue in most cases when the drugs are tailed off.

Different preventive drugs have been tried in the past but, with recent advances, have been superseded by more effective medication. They are mentioned here because they are sometimes prescribed in special circumstances.

Beta-blockers

Both adrenaline and noradrenaline play a part in the production of migraine, as they are produced by stress and affect the reactivity of blood vessels. This 'beta' action of adrenaline and noradrenaline (beta-adrenergic effects) can be countered by a group of drugs called beta-blockers. In small doses these act mainly outside the brain but can calm symptoms of trembling and anxiety, and lower a rapid pulse rate. Because beta-adrenergic

Table 9.2 Drugs to prevent migraine

Beta-blockers	atenolol metoprolol nadolol propranolol timolol
Serotonin antagonists	methysergide (used with caution) pizotifen
Calcium blockers	flunarizine (not licensed in the UK for migraine) nimodipine verapamil
Antidepressants	tricyclics (e.g. amitriptyline) monoamine oxidase inhibitors (MAOIs) selective serotonin re-uptake inhibitors (SSRIs) tetracyclics
Anti-epileptic drugs	gabapentin topiramate valproate
Tranquillisers	benzodiazepines: chlordiazepoxide (Librium), clonazepam (Rivotril), diazepam (Valium), lorazepam (Ativan)
Others	botulinum toxin clonidine magnesium pain-killers (e.g. NSAIDs) vitamins (e.g. riboflavin)

effects are of importance in migraine, beta-blockers help prevent attacks and are the preferred treatment, particularly for people with raised blood pressure. Not all beta-blockers work in migraine so beta-blockade may not be the explanation of their anti-migraine effect.

The prevention of migraine by beta-blockers was a chance finding when propranolol, given to people who had angina as well as migraine, was found to help both conditions. The dose should be the least necessary to prevent attacks; it varies from 40 to 240mg daily. Up to 80 per cent of those using it have achieved a reduction in the frequency of attacks by over 50 per cent. The most common side-effect is fatigue – physical rather than mental. Insomnia and vivid dreams may occur, in which case other beta-blockers (e.g. metoprolol and atenolol) can be used. Slowing of the pulse and lowering blood pressure are not significant unless they produce symptoms such as faintness or dizziness on standing up.

The time taken for half of the amount of drug taken to disappear from the body is known as its half-life; nadolol has a long half-life and can be taken once a day. The half-life of propranolol is about six hours so it can be taken twice a day but there is also a long-acting preparation that can be taken once a day.

Not all beta-blockers are effective for migraine but those that are include atenolol, metoprolol and timolol.

Serotonin antagonists

Pizotifen
A drug that was once widely used is pizotifen (Sanomigran) – a powerful anti-5-HT agent, as well as an antihistamine. One study found that, after taking the standard dose of three tablets a day (1.5mg) for two weeks, about 80 per cent of people noticed that they had fewer migraine headaches; other studies, however, were not so positive. Pizotifen also has a mild antidepressant effect, and another benefit is that coexisting allergies improve as well.

Yvor Zandar, a 27-year-old casualty doctor, began to have severe migraine attacks every week. The headaches would begin behind his right eye, which watered and became red. Instead of the pain lasting a short time – as in cluster headache – there would then follow a severe headache, lasting many hours, accompanied by vomiting. This made it extremely difficult to work the long hours expected and he felt guilty when his friends had to 'cover' for him during a migraine attack. Examination revealed no abnormality and he began to take pizotifen. Within two weeks the headaches stopped and he was able to pass a stiff examination shortly afterwards. He had suffered from hay-fever but reported that, although the pollen count was high, this too had disappeared. After six months the treatment was phased out and the headaches did not return.

Half the people who are helped by pizotifen do not get a recurrence of headaches once treatment has stopped. It is as if the body 'unlearns' its previous pattern of response and no longer produces a migraine attack.

There are two main unwanted effects with pizotifen. The first is drowsiness, so the manufacturers advise care when driving or operating machinery, and suggest that alcohol is not drunk while on this treatment – a caution that also applies to other anti-5-HT, as well as to antihistamine, agents. The other effect is that about one-third of people using it put on weight of the order of about 3kg (7lb), because inhibiting 5 HT in the brain (which happens to a slight extent) increases the appetite. Because of these two effects, pizotifen is no longer in the first-line choice of drugs to prevent migraine.

Methysergide
Probably the most effective anti-serotonin preventive is methysergide. It is often asked why such a drug (i.e. a 5-HT antagonist) works as a preventive whereas the best treatment for acute attacks are triptans, which support the action of serotonin (i.e. 5-HT agonists). The answer is that there are many different types of 5-HT receptors in the brain and that preventive and acute treatments act on these different types.

The reason why methysergide is not a first-choice drug is its side-effects. Quite apart from its milder gastrointestinal effects, which include indigestion and nausea, it can cause muscle pains, especially when walking. The more serious side-effect is the formation of fibrous (scar) tissue in the body, particularly around the kidneys, which can cause kidney failure. Fortunately, this side-effect can be prevented if there is a month's break in treatment every few months (not more than six months). The month's 'holiday' may be trying because of withdrawal symptoms but they can be prevented by a weaning period of one week out of the month.

Precautionary investigations to detect the onset of this scarring include an erythrocyte sedimentation rate (ESR), which will be raised early on, MRI of the abdomen, echocardiography and chest X-ray.

Methysergide should not be taken by anyone with a vascular or cardiac problem.

Calcium blockers

These agents (also called calcium channel blockers) are so named because they prevent the entry of calcium into the cells of muscle in the walls of blood vessels and nerve cells. Flunarizine, used more on the European continent than in the UK, is effective in a dose of 10mg at bedtime. Its most prominent side-effects include weight gain and drowsiness.

Nimodipine and verapamil are occasionally effective in preventing migraine but are not generally the drugs of first choice.

Antidepressants

Depression is divided into *primary* (endogenous), where there is no obvious cause, and *secondary* (exogenous), which is a reaction to untoward circumstances. If psychological techniques are unavailing, depression is easily helped with antidepressant drugs. Of the three main types, the most commonly used are the *tricyclics*, such as amitriptyline. It works by increasing the level of noradrenaline in the brain and thus controls mood. Because the drug accumulates in the blood, it may take up to two weeks before its antidepressant effect is noticed. Common side-effects are dryness of the mouth, blurring of vision or alteration in the heart rate.

Although amitriptyline is listed as an antidepressant, it acts in this way when given in larger doses of more than 150mg per day. In smaller doses of 10–25mg it is given for its action against headache. It is highly effective and the 'drug of choice' for tension-type headache and when both this and migraine headache are present, taken either alone or in combination with beta-blockers such as propranolol.

The tricyclics are surprisingly effective against migraine, even in people who are not depressed, because of their anti-serotonin effect. If the migraine is aggravated by depression, or if there is also tension-type (muscle-contraction) headache, treatment with tricyclics is particularly rewarding.

The chief side-effect of the tricyclic antidepressants such as amitriptyline is drowsiness; for this reason it is begun at the lowest dose possible (10mg) given at night, and preferably 1–2 hours before bedtime. Taken this way the sleepiness wears off after the first or second morning. The next most common side-effects are a dry mouth, blurred vision or palpitations (awareness of a rapid heart beat) but none of these is necessarily troublesome. The reason for the possible side-effects is that these drugs act on receptors other than serotonin.

Similar to the tricyclics but with fewer side-effects is the second group of antidepressants, the newer *tetracyclics*. They are not as effective in migraine but they have the advantage that they exert their antidepressant effects almost at once. The more modern antidepressants such as the selective serotonin re uptake inhibitors (SSRIs) are not as effective against headache and are given more to treat associated depression.

The third group of antidepressants act as inhibitors of the enzyme monoamine oxidase (MAO) – *monoamine oxidase inhibitors*. (MAO breaks down amines, substances that play a part in transmitting nervous impulses – neurotransmitters.) MAO inhibitors are also effective in treating people with migraine, and not just those who are depressed. This is surprising because the level of MAO is low during an attack of migraine, but there are several forms of MAO, and inhibitors may act on only one variety. People taking MAO inhibitors should not eat food containing tyramine (such as cheese), as they may develop reactions such as episodes of high blood pressure. The use of these drugs is limited to more serious cases of depression and they are best avoided for migraine, not least because they have interactions with migraine treatments such as Midrid.

Tranquillisers

The most common predisposing conditions in migraine are stress, anxiety or tension. If these are not relieved by psycho-therapeutic means, there are several tranquillising drugs that can help and thus prevent migraine attacks. The most widely used group of tranquillisers are the *benzodiazepines*, of which diazepam (Valium) and chlordiazepoxide (Librium) are the best known. However, they are best avoided except for occasional use. First introduced to treat epilepsy, clonazepam has been used in migraine but is best avoided because of its habituating effect.

Tranquillising drugs exert a calming effect by acting on the parts of the brain concerned with emotion. (Apart from this effect on the specific receptors in the brain, diazepam relaxes muscle, which, although helpful in muscle-contraction headaches, may produce habituation.) The soothing effect of these drugs on anxiety or agitation also makes people less likely to react to external stress, so it can be very effective in reducing the frequency of headaches. Small doses are prescribed to prevent untoward side-effects such as drowsiness; other unwanted effects of diazepam, such as depression, apathy and loss of muscle tone, are also avoided by taking low doses. If they are taken in high dosage for long periods, there may be more serious side-effects – for example, personality changes such as sudden rages and irritability similar to those experienced with other forms of addiction (e.g. alcohol, LSD). Other benzodiazepines include lorazepam (Ativan) and chlordiazepoxide (Librium).

Stopping taking these tranquillisers should be done gradually, because doing it suddenly can result in episodes of anxiety.

Anti-epileptic drugs

Nearly all of these have been tried in the treatment of migraine. More recently, gabapentin, topiramate and valproate have survived, with some success, the requirements of scientifically proven clinical trials. Topiramate has been effective in some patients.

Other preventive drugs

Clonidine
The first agent given to prevent migraine was clonidine, first used to treat high blood pressure and acts both on the brain and on blood vessels. Centres in the brain that control blood pressure are affected in such a way that they cause blood vessels to dilate, while the blood vessels themselves are made less responsive to noradrenaline; both of these actions serve to reduce blood pressure. In smaller doses, clonidine should prevent many of the

chemical changes that spark off a migraine attack; Dixarit, its trade name, contains about a quarter of the dose of clonidine used for high blood pressure. When it prevents migraine in this dosage, it works well, but people who do not benefit from initial treatment will not benefit from a higher dosage.

A group of medical students were given either clonidine or a placebo before a party in which they consumed an excessive amount of wine and cheese. The next morning the clonidine group developed headache significantly less often than the group who took the placebo. This result, although not scientifically reported, is interesting because red wine and cheese is often reported as a trigger in producing headaches. The 'hangover' headache is due to a variety of factors, one of which is that the alcohol dehydrates the brain tissue to give low-pressure headache (see Chapter 2). Some of the chemicals in alcoholic drinks have effects on their own, acting to cause a migraine type headache. The part that an excess of tobacco plays in the hangover headache is uncertain but nicotine can be a precipitant of headache.

Although several trials have found that clonidine is of no benefit when compared with a placebo, it can be useful in certain circumstances, because of its almost total lack of side-effects, especially in women whose migraine attacks occur at the time of their menstrual periods. Like other preventive drugs, it may take up to two weeks for it to have any effect. It is seldom prescribed nowadays.

Botulinum toxin

There has been much in the press recently about the use of botulinum toxin type A (Botox). Botulinum toxin is the purified toxin from the bacterium *Clostridium botulinum*, which is found in rotting vegetable matter. The bacterium has been the cause of outbreaks of botulism in which people who eat tainted food develop paralysis, can no longer breathe and may even die. The toxin has an effect of irreversibly blocking the connections between the nerves and the muscles, thus paralysing them. Eventually, the connections regrow but this takes about three months. Botulinum toxin also works by blocking the release of inflammatory substances from sensory neurones.

Botulinum toxin was first used medically in the field of ophthalmology to control double vision (diplopia) due to squint (strabismus). Strabismus is caused by an imbalance in the muscles that move the eyes when one eye moves more than the other, causing double vision. Injection of an extremely dilute solution of botulinum toxin can cause weakness in one of the stronger muscles and thus restore the balance.

Since the 1980s botulinum toxin has been used in the treatment of many other disorders. They include abnormal twitching of the face, painful spasm of the neck or back muscles and spasticity (e.g. cerebral palsy). More recently it has been used in plastic surgery to eradicate wrinkles, which are caused by contractions in muscles attached beneath the skin. Injection of these muscles with botulinum toxin relaxes the muscles and eradicates the wrinkles for about three months, whereupon the procedure has to be repeated. Many cosmetic surgeons have been using botulinum toxin, and its use is increasing.

A fortuitous discovery was that some people with migraine whose wrinkles had been treated with botulinum experienced an improvement in the frequency and the severity of their headaches. Botulinum toxin type A has reduced the frequency and severity of attacks in some people with migraine better than a placebo. Studies show that it is more effective in people with frequent migraine headaches and in those with spasm in the neck muscles (e.g. following a car accident).

Botulinum toxin has been helpful in a number of people, usually those with typical migraine symptoms, but is still undergoing clinical trials in some European countries, with a similar trial in the USA. The results will not be available before the end of 2004.

Using botulinum toxin to treat migraine is still in an early phase from the scientific point of view but many doctors are beginning to use it 'off licence' (or 'off label'). 'Off licence' means that the drug is being used for a purpose other than that for which it was licensed. This is perfectly acceptable provided the doctor accepts the responsibility and the patient agrees after being fully informed. The manufacturer of the medication is forbidden by law to advertise any 'off licence' usage. Over 1 million people have been treated for various conditions and there is little in the way of side-effects. Treatment needs to be given every three months because the effect of the drug wears off. It can involve up to 20 injections, which can be painful.

Pain-killers

Aspirin is the most common pain reliever and nearly everyone has taken this drug. It acts by preventing the formation of prostaglandin, a naturally occurring fatty substance with a wide variety of actions. Other drugs also work in this way; they include a variety of anti-rheumatics such as ibuprofen and indometacin. Many people with migraine respond well, the headaches being less intense and less frequent when these drugs are used as preventives. It is best to use them in the lowest dose possible, because with higher doses side-effects may occur: indigestion and, particularly in people with a history of indigestion or peptic ulcer, actual bleeding in the stomach.

Magnesium

Although claims have been made for the efficacy of magnesium in preventing migraine attacks, and no consistent scientific evidence has confirmed these, there have been encouraging studies.

Vitamins

Various vitamins have been tried but the only one proved to be effective in clinical trials is vitamin B_2, although there is some evidence for vitamin B_6.

Conclusion

The success of preventive (prophylactic) medication depends on the dose and timing. The drug is usually begun at a relatively small dose, increasing gradually until it is effective or there are unacceptable side-effects. They should be used for three to six weeks before increasing the dose or changing to another migraine prophylactic.

The main difficulty is that, as the migraine attacks become less of a problem, it is difficult to persuade people to take the medication regularly. The aim is to completely prevent attacks. If this is successful, the longer the period of freedom from attacks, the more likely is this improvement to continue when the drug is stopped.

10
Headache clinics and the future

Headache clinics

The realisation that migraine – one of the most common causes of headache – is a disorder causing a vast amount of unnecessary suffering has led to great interest in the subject, much increased by the discovery of more effective drugs for preventing and, particularly, for treating migraine attacks. Although specialist centres have been set up for the treatment of acute migraine attacks, there are not enough for all the people who need treatment and advice, particularly without a letter of referral from their GP.

A headache clinic is a patient-care system devoted to diagnosing and treating head pain. Typically staffed by multidisciplinary teams that include neurologists and psychologists, these clinics offer specialised services for people with difficult headache problems. They may offer a range of diagnostic services from electroencephalography to neuro-imaging procedures such as MRI on-site. Headache clinics are not widely available, and most people will initially consult their family doctor; less than 5 per cent would be referred to a neurologist and even fewer to one specialising in headache and migraine.

The main reasons someone is referred to a headache clinic are:

- The diagnosis is in doubt after evaluation by a non-specialist. Specialisation increases expertise, so a doctor concentrating on people with headaches becomes more knowledgeable about the possible causes; this is particularly important when previous efforts at treatment of rare disorders have been unsuccessful.
- Response to treatment is not satisfactory.

- A change in frequency of the headache due to:
  - daily headaches from medication overuse or rebound;
  - other medical conditions complicating management.

Once the diagnosis of migraine is made, a plan for preventing attacks and for treating acute attacks will be developed.

Perhaps the most important function of the headache clinic is to deal with and study attacks, which, surprisingly, are rarely seen by most hospital doctors. In such clinics, tests are performed on people with a migraine attack, which give a better idea of what happens during an attack – for example, that the stomach muscle does not contract (gastric stasis) and medications do not work because they are not passed on to the small intestine where they are absorbed. This explains why drugs work only when taken at the beginning of an attack, before gastric stasis occurs.

The insight thus gained has helped in the development of more appropriate treatment, such as metoclopramide (Maxolon), which counteracts gastric stasis. This was revealed by measuring the levels in the blood of aspirin taken during an attack. The finding that the levels were lower than when aspirin was taken at other times confirmed that stomach emptying was slow during an attack, resulting in the recommendation to use metoclopramide to stimulate the gut and aid absorption.

The advantage of grouping together people with the same disorder is that it allows the clinic staff to acquire greater experience and expertise in that specialised area, thus helping find effective treatments. It also facilitates research into the disorder.

The ideal clinic

The ideal headache clinic has a neurologist in attendance, because the causes of headache not due to migraine need to be determined. Investigative facilities for this are required, in addition to facilities for more elaborate tests that might be needed. A clinical pharmacologist (an expert in the use of drugs) should be available to advise on dosage and administration of drugs and on the setting up of clinical trials of new medication.

In a sleep laboratory, an individual is in a single room and can be assessed using laboratory apparatus such as an electro-encephalograph (EEG) machine to monitor changes occurring during sleep. By EEG monitoring from leads attached to the person's head, researchers are able to see which stage of sleep has been reached. Such research has led to the finding that the levels of noradrenaline in people who have early-morning migraine rise one to two hours before they wake up – generally from REM (rapid eye movement) sleep. REM sleep is so called because in this stage there are rapid eye movements, and dreaming occurs. These periods happen about four times a night, each one lasting about 20 minutes. During dreaming the body responds just as it does during the same real activities; for example, running for a bus in a dream causes the heart to beat faster and this is associated with a rise in noradrenaline levels. The rise in noradrenaline levels before an early-morning migraine may be related to dreams caused by stresses during waking life.

It must be emphasised that few NHS headache or migraine clinics have these facilities. Headache clinics are expensive. For example:

- some blood tests can cost up to £50,
- an EEG machine can cost over £10,000, each EEG test costing about £200,
- an MRI machine costs over £500,000, each scan costing over £600.

No matter how high these costs are, however, they are more than offset by saving costs to the economy through time lost from work.

Headache associations

As with many other disorders, people with migraine have formed support groups – for example, the Migraine Trust and the Migraine Action Association in the UK (details in the 'Useful addresses' section at the back of this book), and the National Migraine Foundation in the USA.

There are many such headache support groups around the world who have joined in an international organisation called the World Headache Alliance. This is a collaboration whose aim is to further the cause of headache patients and headache associations across the world and to increase their visibility allowing them to raise more funds for services and research. The International Headache Society was founded in 1987 and is composed of physicians and researchers interested in the subject of headache. Every two years they hold a meeting which is extremely well attended and the proceedings are published in its journal *Cephalalgia*. There is also a European Headache Society that meets regularly, in different European countries, mainly for educational purposes. The World Federation of Neurology has sessions on headache, as does the American Academy of Neurology and other national neurological associations.

The future

The nature of migraine

There is evidence indicating that there are differences between people who have migraine and those who do not. The cause of the episodic nature of attacks is not known but some people wake up and know that they will have a migraine on that day. On what does this fluctuating tendency depend? The cause of these fluctuations could be 'biological clocks' that affect the cycles of hormones; in women, the menstrual cycle is one obvious example.

Research funds

There is no doubt that a number of people from different disciplines working on the same problem, with sufficient funds, can do a lot more in research than separate groups working independently. This is easier to fund where salaries are comparatively low, which is why multi-national pharmaceutical companies may do much of their basic research in particular countries.

New drugs

The migraine attack is now readily treatable, but more work is needed on compounds taken by mouth that are absorbed quickly and act quickly and effectively. Using drugs to prevent an attack (prophylaxis) is now common but more effective preventives are needed. Any drug is, at most, 80 per cent effective; this leaves 20 per cent of people still needing help, and a wider choice of different medications would be useful.

Because of side-effects, it is undesirable to use drugs to treat what is in effect a life-long problem. Interest in non-drug techniques – for example, using biofeedback and methods that enable the people to control their own bodily functions – is continuing to increase, particularly because migraine, like high blood pressure, would seem to lend itself well to this sort of approach.

Scientific 'breakthroughs' are exceptional and are, in spite of the name, usually the result of slowly built-up theories. The same applies to the development of new treatments. There may be hundreds of similar compounds capable of helping people with migraine but each must first be tested in animals for effectiveness and for side-effects. A compound may have too weak or too short-lived an effect. The search can go on for years, and, when a promising compound is found, toxicity studies need to be undertaken, again first in animals. Any profound side-effect can lead to its rejection, even after work done for many years.

Once toxicity studies have ended, pilot studies in human volunteers can be undertaken, again to determine the compound's effectiveness and any side-effects. These trials have to be approved by the government Committee for the Safety of Medicines. After this come large-scale drug trials and only then general release of the drug. All these processes can take up to 20 years, so it is amazingly expensive for a pharmaceutical company to produce a new drug. It has been suggested that the cost of putting a drug on the market from its discovery is over £100,000,000.

People with migraine respond differently to hormonal stress, possibly due to the chemical messengers differing in reactivity. The attack itself poses many questions. Why, for instance, does there seem to be a cycle that in some people has to run its full length? In these people, drugs only delay the ending, making the symptoms drag on for days. It is not known why this abnormality persists but it is more potent than some of our strongest drugs. It is to be hoped that further research will solve these problems and the many others concerned with one of the most common afflictions of humans.

Appendix
Relaxation exercises

General introduction

The therapist should make sure that you are comfortable and supported. The theory of relaxation is explained, as is the need for relaxation. This is followed by a short explanation of the system used and examples of the best method to follow – with the reassurance that it is easy and individually tailored. Once the routine has been learned, you can continue the exercises regularly at home.

Contraction and relaxation exercises

Lie on your back on the floor, with your head on a pillow.

- Tense your whole body (leg muscles, stomach muscles, facial muscles, etc.) and relax

- Take a deep breath in and let it out with a sigh

- Repeat once

- Tense your left leg, raising it slightly off the floor – feel the tension throughout your leg (in your ankle, calf, knee, thigh)

- Feel discomfort . . . and relax

- Feel that the leg is heavy on the floor, heavy and relaxed

- Repeat with your right leg

- Now let the floor take all the weight of your legs. There should be no more tension – they are completely relaxed

- Hunch your shoulders up to your ears – feel the tension down your spine, across your back, in your neck
- Relax

- Tense your left arm, raising it slightly off the ground
- Clench your fist, tighten and rotate your wrist – feel the tension in your forearm, your elbow, and upper arm
- Relax
- Let your arm rest heavily on the floor, completely relaxed
- Repeat with your right arm

There should be no more tension in your arms or your legs. The floor should take all their weight, heavy and relaxed.

- Raise your head off the pillow and turn it as far to the left as possible
- Now to the right – feeling the tension
- Back to the centre and let your head fall on to the pillow – heavy and relaxed

There should be no tension in your neck at all. Your head is resting heavily on the pillow.

- Take a deep breath in and let it out with a sigh

- Now tense the muscle of your buttocks – pull in as hard as you can
- Relax

- Arch your back off the floor slightly – feel the contraction and tension right through your spine
- Relax
- Take a deep breath in and let it out with a long sigh

- Now tense your stomach – pull in the muscles so hard that you can feel the tension in your chest as well

- Hold it till it almost hurts

- Relax

- Take another deep breath in and let it out with a long sigh

Your whole body should now be completely supported by the floor. There is no tension anywhere, no discomfort. You feel pleasantly heavy and relaxed.

Now relax your facial muscles.

- First frown as hard as you can, drawing your brows as close together as possible

- Relax   feel your forehead smoothing out

- Screw up your eyes as tightly as possible – feel the discomfort

- Relax

- Leave your eyelids slightly closed – feel your eyes heavy in their sockets . . . heavy and relaxed

- Clench your jaw and push your tongue against your lower teeth – feel the discomfort of tension

- Relax – let your jaw drop slightly and your tongue drop behind your lower teeth

Feel all your facial muscles smooth and relaxed.

Suggestion therapy or autohypnosis

The second part of the exercise outlined above follows.
Say to yourself:

- I feel my legs growing heavier and heavier and more

relaxed. There is no tension right through from my ankles to my hips. Heavy and relaxed.

■ I feel my arms growing heavier and heavier. My hands are heavy, wrists are loose. The floor takes all their weight.

■ My head is heavy on the pillow, heavy and relaxed. There is no tension down my spine or across my shoulders. My whole body is relaxed and supported.

■ My forehead feels broad and smooth. The space between my eyes seems very wide, and all tension around my eyes and round my mouth has gone.

■ My jaw is relaxed. All my facial muscles are at rest, relaxed. I am completely relaxed. And while my body is relaxed, I try to let my mind relax, too.

Glossary

Words given in *italic* in the definitions are also defined in this Glossary.

acetylcholine a chemical acting at the junction between nerves and muscles, and in the *parasympathetic nervous system* (see also *neurotransmitter*)

acute in the context of migraine, this refers to a short-term attack or its treatment (see also *chronic*)

allergy abnormal reaction by the body's immune system to a 'foreign' substance

analgesic a pain-killing drug

anecdotal informal reports or comments, as opposed to reports from formal studies or research

aura this term is used to describe the symptoms of an impending attack of either migraine or epilepsy

benzodiazepines a group of drugs used as tranquillisers, e.g. diazepam (Valium), nitrazepam (Mogadon), flurazepam (Dalmane)

beta-receptor one of the body's receptors stimulated by adrenaline

biochemistry the study of the chemical reactions that take place in the body (literally: the chemistry of life)

biofeedback the term for relaying back information, usually into the conscious mind, regarding an automatic function. With this technique it is hoped that these unconscious processes can be brought under 'voluntary control' – using an electro-myograph (EMG), muscle contraction can be seen and the individual can learn, by watching the monitor, to relax.

cerebrospinal fluid (CSF) the fluid that bathes the brain and spinal cord

chronic in a medical context, this means long-term or long-lasting

123

computed tomography (CT) an imaging system that uses X-rays

cortex the grey matter that forms the outer part of the brain substance

cranial nerves the twelve pairs of nerves that arise from the brain itself. Their functions are:

I	smell
II	vision
III, IV and VI	eye movements
V	sensation of face, chewing
VII	facial muscles
VIII	hearing and balance
IX	movement of the palate, taste
X	function of the parasympathetic nervous system
XI	some shoulder muscles
XII	tongue movements

CT see *computed tomography*

electroencephalography (EEG) the recording of the electrical activity of the brain

electromyography (EMG) the recording of the electrical activity of muscles and the speed of transmission of a nerve impulse

endorphins the body's natural pain-killers

enzyme a biological substance that speeds up chemical reactions

epilepsy an epileptic attack is caused by abnormal electrical activity in the brain and consists of either involuntary movements of the body or loss of consciousness. It can be either inherited or acquired due to a structural abnormality of the brain (e g. stroke, tumour or brain damage)

erythrocyte sedimentation rate (ESR) a blood test that measures the rate of fall in a tube of the red blood cells (erythrocytes); it aids in the diagnosis of inflammation

familial a tendency for diseases or conditions to run in families

frontal lobe the front part of each cerebral *hemisphere*

hemianopia blindness of half of a *visual field*

hemisphere one side of the brain

hormone a chemical substance that controls certain functions of the body

immunology the study of the body's defence systems against foreign proteins such as germs (micro-organisms). White blood cells are of two types: one, called lymphocytes, produces

antibodies that cause foreign substances to be cleared from
the circulation or make them more likely to be engulfed by
the second type, called polymorphs, which act as scavengers.
An inappropriate immune response can damage the body
(*allergy*)

ischaemia lack of blood to a body tissue

kinin a chemical substance that, among other actions, may
increase pain and is associated with inflammatory activity

lithium a light metal, whose 'salt' is used as a tranquilliser,
particularly in dampening mood swings. It is also used in the
treatment of *chronic* cluster headache

magnetic resonance imaging (MRI) a type of imaging system
that uses magnetic fields

monosodium glutamate a substance used to increase the
flavouring of foods (found especially in Chinese cuisine)

MRI see *magnetic resonance imaging*

neurone a nerve cell

neurophysiology the study of the way the nervous system works

neurotransmitter a chemical that passes an impulse between
two adjoining nerve cells (*synapse*)

occipital lobe the back part of the brain, concerned with vision

parasympathetic nervous system one of the two parts of the
'autonomic' nervous system. *Acetylcholine* is the main *neurotransmitter* used. Activation of this system causes, among
other changes, the heart to slow and the pupils to constrict.
(See also *sympathetic nervous system.*)

parietal lobe the area of the cerebral *hemisphere* midway
between the *frontal* and *occipital* areas

phonophobia a dislike of noise

photophobia a dislike of light

physiology the study of the how the body is organised and works

placebo a 'dummy' substance given instead of a drug. Although
the help that a placebo has given (particularly for pain) was
previously thought to be due to suggestion, recent work
suggests that there may be an activation of *endorphins*

platelet a very small blood cell that plays an important part in
clotting; it stores many chemical substances, including 5-HT

prostacyclin a derivative of arachidonic acid, produced by the
vessel wall; although very short-lived, it has potent anti-
clotting and *vasodilating* actions

prophylactic a substance used to prevent an attack or condition

referred pain pain that is felt to be somewhere in the body other than where it actually occurs

scotoma a blind spot in the *visual field*

stroke a disturbance of the brain due to either blockage or rupture of a blood vessel

sympathetic nervous system one of the two parts of the 'autonomic' system. The main neurotransmitter is noradrenaline. Activation of the sympathetic nervous system causes an increase in heart rate and a widening of the pupils. (See also *parasympathetic nervous system*.)

synapse the space between two nerve cells (neurones). Nervous impulses are transmitted across the gap by release of chemicals called *neurotransmitters*

temporal arteritis (cranial arteritis) an inflammatory condition of blood vessels, characterised by severe continuous headache; it occurs only in elderly people

temporal lobe the part of the brain next to the *parietal* and *occipital* lobes

tricyclics a class of antidepressant drug (so called because their basic chemical structure consists of three rings)

trigeminal nerve the fifth cranial nerve; literally 'three twins' because it has three divisions – ophthalmic, maxillary and mandibular

ventricles normal cavities in the brain containing *cerebrospinal fluid*

vasoconstriction constriction (narrowing) of a blood vessel

vasodilation expansion, or widening, of the diameter of a blood vessel

visual field the area you can see

Useful addresses

Alexander Technique
see Society of Teachers of the
Alexander Technique

Migraine Action Association
(formerly **British Migraine
Association**)
Unit 6
Oakley Hay Lodge Business Park
Great Folds Road
Great Oakley
Northants NN18 9AS
Tel: 01536 461 333
Fax: 01536 461 444
Website: www.migraine.org.uk
*Founded in 1958, provides
information and support for people
with migraine and their families. Also
raises general awareness of the
condition with workplace seminars,
local meetings and liaison with the
media. Migraine Awareness Week is
held during the first week of
September. The Association also
provides funding for specialist
migraine clinics and patient-focused
research projects.*

Migraine Trust
2nd floor
55–56 Russell Square
London
WC1B 4HP
Tel: 020 7436 1336
Fax: 020 7436 2880
Website: www.migrainetrust.org
*Founded in 1965, this is a charitable
body that distributes information
about migraine in the form of a
newsletter, a paperback on migraine,
a letter-answering service and support
of research throughout the UK, and
the rest of the world if funds are
available. Every two years the Trust
organises an International Migraine
Symposium at which experts from all
over the world gather; the report of
their research activities into all
aspects of the migraine problem is
then published. The money to fund
these activities is raised from private
donations and fund-raising activities.*
Mission statement: 'The Migraine
Trust seeks to empower migraine
sufferers through information and
support whilst educating health
professionals and actively funding
and disseminating research.'

**Society of Teachers
of the Alexander Technique**
1st floor
Linton House
39–51 Highgate Road
London
NW5 1RS
Tel: 020 7284 3338
Fax: 020 7482 5435
Website: www.stat.org.uk
*For general information and lists of
teachers of the Alexander technique
in the UK and world-wide, and
recommended training schools.*

Bandolier website
www.ebandolier.com
*An e-journal with the latest evidence-
based research data on a wide variety
of subjects. Written for doctors, so
quite technical, but deliberately aims
at being very readable.*

Index

Have you found *Migraine: Practical advice to help you manage your migraine* useful and practical? If so, you may be interested in other books from Class Publishing.

Allergies – the 'at your fingertips' guide £14.99
Dr Joanne Clough
This authoritative handbook covers a broad range of allergies, including asthma, eczema, dermatitis and hay-fever, and anaphylaxis, and gives you clear and concise information on allergies – what they are, how they develop, and most importantly, how to deal with them.

> "Extremely enjoyable and informative." – Susan Ollier, Scientific Director, British Allergy Foundation

High Blood Pressure – the 'at your fingertips' guide
NEW THIRD EDITION
DUE IN JANUARY 2004
£14.99
Professor Tom Fahey,
Professor Deirdre Murphy
with Dr Julian Tudor Hart
The authors use all their years of experience as blood pressure experts to answer over 340 real questions on high blood pressure, including questions you may feel uneasy about asking your doctor, as well as offering positive, practical advice on every aspect of your blood pressure.

> "... an excellent book, with a comprehensive questions and answer format which will solve any query." – Dr Donald McKendrick, Saga Magazine

Cancer – the 'at your fingertips' guide
THIRD EDITION £14.99
Val Speechley and Maxine Rosenfield
This invaluable reference guide gives you clear and practical information about cancer. Whether you have cancer yourself or are caring for someone who does, you will find in this book the information you need to reassure yourself, and enable you to take control.

Food Allergies: Enjoying life with a severe food allergy £14.99
Tanya Wright
Expert dietitian Tanya Wright combines her professional and personal experience of severe food allergy to give you a unique source of practical advice. She guides you carefully through the different types of food allergy, discussing food labelling and how to prevent anaphylactic reactions.

> "Required reading for those with food allergies." – David Reading, Director, The Anaphylaxis Campaign

Heart Health – the 'at your fingertips' guide
SECOND EDITION £14.99
Dr Graham Jackson
This practical handbook, written by a leading cardiologist, answers all your questions about heart conditions. It tells you all about you and your heart; how to keep your heart healthy – or, if it has been affected by heart disease, how to make it as strong as possible.

> "... answers the questions in a way that the doctor wishes he had given, if only he had the time." – Dr Thomas Stuttaford, The Times

Beating Depression – the 'at your fingertips' guide £14.99
Dr Stefan Cembrowicz and Dr Dorcas Kingham
Depression is one of most common illnesses in the world – affecting up to one in four people at some time in their lives. *Beating Depression* shows sufferers and their families that they are not alone, and offers tried and tested techniques for overcoming depression.

> "A sympathetic and understanding guide." – Marjorie Wallace, Chief Executive, SANE

PRIORITY ORDER FORM

Cut out or photocopy this form and send it
(post free in the UK) to.

Class Publishing (Priority Service)
FREEPOST
London W6 7BR

Please send me urgently   *Post included*
(*enter quantity below*)   *price per copy*
                                                        (UK only)

☐ *Migraine: Practical advice to help you manage*   £17.99
   your migraine (ISBN 1 85959 066 7)

☐ *Allergies – the 'at your fingertips' guide*   £17.99
   (ISBN 1 872362 52 4)

☐ *Food Allergies: Enjoying life with a severe food allergy*   £17.99
   (ISBN 1 85959 039 X)

☐ *High Blood Pressure – the 'at your fingertips' guide*   £17.99
   (ISBN 1 85959 090 X)

☐ *Heart Health – the 'at your fingertips' guide*   £17.99
   (ISBN 1 85959 009 8)

☐ *Cancer – the 'at your fingertips' guide*   £17.99
   (ISBN 1 85959 036 5)

☐ *Beating Depression – the 'at your fingertips' guide*   £17.99
   (ISBN 1 85959 063 2)

                                        Total   _____

EASY WAYS TO PAY

Cheque: I enclose a cheque payable to Class Publishing for _____

Credit card: Please debit my Mastercard ☐ Visa ☐ Amex ☐ Switch ☐

Card no. _____ Expiry date _____

Name _____

Delivery address _____

_____

Town _____ Postcode _____

Daytime telephone (*in case of query*) _____

Credit card billing address (*if different from above*) _____

_____

Town _____ Postcode _____

Class Publishing's guarantee: remember that if, for any reason, you are not satisfied with these books,
we will refund all your money, without any questions asked.
Prices and VAT rates may be altered for reasons beyond our control.

The 'at your fingertips' series

Our best selling series, the *at your fingertips* guides seek to help those who, having been diagnosed with a condition, have countless questions that need answering. These essential handbooks answer all the questions that patients want to know about their health and condition. The formula for the series follows a question-and-answer format, with real questions from sufferers and their families answered by medical experts at the top of their fields, without the jargon of medical texts. All these books are packed full of practical information for patients and their families. Each title is only £14.99 plus p&p. Topics covered range from diagnosis to treatment, and from relationships to welfare entitlements.

Titles currently available (or coming soon*):

Acne • Allergies • Asthma • Autism* • Beating Depression Cancer • COPD* • Dementia – Alzheimer's & other dementias Diabetes • Epilepsy • Eczema* • Gout • Heart Health High Blood Pressure • Kidney Dialysis & Transplants Motor Neurone Disease • Multiple Sclerosis • Osteoporosis* Parkinson's • Psoriasis • Sexual Health for Men • Stroke

For current availability of the *at your fingertips* range, please contact us using our Freepost address:

**Class Publishing Priority Service
FREEPOST
London W6 7BR**

The *Class Health* Feedback Form

We hope that you found this *Class Health* book helpful. We always appreciate readers' opinions and would be grateful if you could take a few minutes to complete this form for us.

1 **How did you acquire your copy of this book?**

From my local library ☐

Read an article in a newspaper/magazine ☐

Found it by chance ☐

Recommended by a friend ☐

Recommended by a patient organisation/charity ☐

Recommended by a doctor/nurse/advisor ☐

Saw an advertisement ☐

2 **How much of the book have you read?**

All of it ☐

More than half of it ☐

Less than half of it ☐

3 **Which copies/chapters have been most helpful?**

....

....

4 **Overall, how useful to you was this *Class Health* book?**

Extremely useful ☐

Very useful ☐

Useful ☐

5 **What did you find most helpful?**

....

....

6 **What did you find least helpful?**

....

....

❼ Have you read any other health books?

Yes ☐   No ☐

If yes, which subjects did they cover?

....

....

How did this *Class Health* book compare?

Much better ☐

Better ☐

About the same ☐

Not as good ☐

❽ Would you recommend this book to a friend?

Yes ☐   No ☐

Thank you for your help. Please send your completed form to:

Class Publishing, FREEPOST, London W6 7BR

Surname _____   First name _____

Title Prof/Dr/Mr/Mrs/Ms _____

Address _____

_____

Town _____   Postcode _____

Country _____

☐ Please add my name and address to receive details of related books

  [*Please note, we will not pass on your details to any other company*]

(MIGRAINE 2004)